Praise for *Love and Laughter in the Time of Chemotherapy*:

"By turns heartbreaking, uplifting, witty and wise. A profound and inspiring testament to the power of love, beautifully written by a woman of extraordinary gifts, and I don't just mean writerly gifts. We should all aspire to confront life's challenges with the wisdom, grace, humour and, yes, love, that guide Manjusha Pawagi on her journey. She is a wonder, and so is this book."
—TERRY FALLIS, two-time winner of the Stephen Leacock Memorial Medal for Humour for *Best Laid Plans* and *No Relation*

"Manjusha Pawagi carries us on her journey through a territory that is unspeakably rough, with all the humor and grace that any traveller can muster. We learn with her what it feels like to be knocked off-course in the prime of life, and to work one's way back. *Love and Laughter in the Time of Chemotherapy* is touching, funny, and a privilege to read."
—DANIELLE MARTIN, MD. Author of *Better Now: Six Big Ideas to Improve Health Care for All Canadians*

"Courage. Honesty. Wit. These are the qualities that distinguish Manjusha Pawagi, both as a person, and a writer. *Love and Laughter in the Time of Chemotherapy* is a moving demonstration of this character, in life and in prose."
—ANDREW PYPER, author of *The Only Child*, *Lost Girls*, *The Killing Circle*, and *The Guardians*

LOVE AND LAUGHTER
IN THE TIME OF CHEMOTHERAPY

Love and Laughter
in the time of
Chemotherapy

MANJUSHA PAWAGI

Second Story Press

Library and Archives Canada Cataloguing in Publication

Pawagi, Manjusha, 1967-, author
Love and laughter in the time of chemotherapy /
by Manjusha Pawagi.

Issued in print and electronic formats.
ISBN 978-1-77260-045-2 (softcover).—
ISBN 978-1-77260-046-9 (EPUB)

1. Pawagi, Manjusha, 1967-. 2. Pawagi, Manjusha, 1967-
—Health. 3. Cancer—Patients—Biography. 4. Authors,
Canadian—Biography. 5. Judges—Canada—Biography. I. Title.

PS8581.A8463Z46 2017   C813'.54   C2017-902904-5

C2017-902905-3

Copyright © 2017 by Manjusha Pawagi

Cover photo © iStockphoto
Editors: Carolyn Jackson, Wendy Thomas
Design: Melissa Kaita
Author photo by Jack Farley

Printed and bound in Canada

*Second Story Press gratefully acknowledges the support of the
Ontario Arts Council and the Canada Council for the Arts for our
publishing program. We acknowledge the financial support of the
Government of Canada through the Canada Book Fund.*

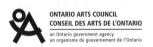

Published by
SECOND STORY PRESS
20 Maud Street, Suite 401
Toronto, ON M5V 2M5
www.secondstorypress.ca

For Jay

Now, I have no choice but to see with your eyes, he said,
so I'm not alone, so you're not alone.

—YIANNIS RITSOS, from the poem, "Maybe, Someday"

I've suffered for my art, now it's your turn.

—STEPHEN FRY, from the novel *The Hippopotamus*

CHAPTER ONE

I USED TO LIE AWAKE at night, planning my husband's funeral. He is not dying. He is not even sick. He did have Hodgkin's lymphoma, but that was when he was an undergraduate student, almost thirty years ago, and he has been in remission ever since. Still, his treatment, as cancer treatments often do, ravaged his body and lungs, and he is prone to getting chest infections. So I worried. If he so much as sneezed, I would picture it as the beginning of the end. I could not stand to think of the loss, so I would concentrate on the actual funeral instead. It made me feel like I had some control. Plus, I like planning things.

And so I'd lie there, glancing occasionally at my clock radio as 3:45 a.m. gave way to 4:17, and then to 5:03, Simon sound asleep beside me. Friends complain about husbands snoring, but I have the opposite issue. I have never known such a silent sleeper. I would have to hold my own breath to catch even the smallest sound of breathing from him, and then I could finally relax. I would worry that I was dreaming him and I'd gently pinch him to make sure he was real.

"If you think you're dreaming," he once said pointedly, "you're supposed to pinch *yourself*, not me."

I always start with the music; all Leonard Cohen, because it is so naturally funereal. But not actually *sung* by Leonard Cohen, because that would be too much. I want to move people, not make them suicidal. I intend to use Toronto torch singer Patricia O'Callaghan, whose covers of Leonard Cohen I have had on constant repeat in my car for six months straight. I'll start with my favorite, "The Window." It's so beautiful that I hit repeat before it finishes because I'm sad at the thought of it ending even before it does (the same way I think about Simon's imminent demise). I'm not sure the cello introduction is long enough, but ideally it will last until people settle down and realize the service is beginning. And then Patricia will start with the words "Why do you stand by the window…"

Next will be "Dance Me to the End of Love" during the slide show. It might be tricky, but I would like to time the photos of Simon and our twins, Jack and Anna, to appear with the line "Dance me to the children who are asking to be born." There's one photo I would save for the little card you give everyone as a memento; it's the one of Simon on the deck of my parents' cottage, tanned and smiling straight at me (since I'm the photographer). He has a baby in each arm; Jack and Anna are about eight months old, their big brown eyes are looking at me solemnly, as only babies can look. Simon's gray eyes are crinkled up by his smile.

"My eyes are sky blue," he corrects me.

I will end with "Hallelujah." I know, I know, you're thinking that is so overdone and obvious, but I've got a surprise in mind. All the boys and girls in the Canadian Children's Opera Company that Anna sings with will be sitting in the balcony in their black and white uniforms. At the chorus, where the word "Hallelujah" is repeated a gazillion times, they will rise to their feet as one and join in with their perfect child voices. The audience will be stunned and amazed and will barely have time to recover before ushers quietly and efficiently distribute handfuls of rose petals, real ones, not fake, for everyone to scatter on the casket (closed).

You're probably wondering, how is she so good at this? (And you may be wondering other things as well.) So I have to reveal that Simon's is not the first death I have anticipated. When I was a child, if my parents returned home even five minutes later than they said they would, I would assume they had been killed by a drunk driver, and that my little brother and I were now orphans. Harish would be there in his pajamas, clutching the board game Aggravation to his chest, begging me to play with him. And I, excellent elder sister/babysitter that I am, would be stationed at the living room window, watching for my parents to turn into our suburban cul-de-sac, and simultaneously running through a mental list of our family friends, looking for potential alternative homes.

Even into my early twenties it continued. I once dated a man who was forty when I was twenty-four. I spent every minute of our time together doing the math. When I'm forty, he'll be fifty-six, so far not too bad. But then when I'm fifty, he'll be sixty-six. And when I'm sixty-five…oh my god, he'll be dead. It didn't matter that it was the kind of relationship you measure in days, not decades; case in point, I once called him only to hang up the second he answered because I only wanted to ascertain that, yes, he had the use of both his phone and his hands and was *choosing* not to call me. I still could not stop fretting about his impending death.

I met Simon on a camping safari in southern Africa in the fall of 1999, going through Zimbabwe, Botswana, and Namibia. He was the only one there from England, I was the only one from Canada. There were others from Germany, the Netherlands, Australia. Two women from the United States, Vicky and Lori, ended up coming to our wedding.

If I try to tell you what we had in common, I'm going to sound stupid: We bought matching wooden giraffes; we had the same favorite Springsteen song, "Thunder Road"; and the same favorite Dickens novel, *Great Expectations*. And since I share my February 7 birthday with Charles Dickens, that last point seemed eerily significant. If I tell you how we were different, you would be alarmed: He barely talks, I barely stop talking; he never worries, I never stop worrying. When I heard him use his inhaler, even way back then, it sounded to me like a death rattle. Yet my doubts were no match for his certainty.

He claims he knew the first time we met, walking in the Kalahari Desert to look at the sunset, but wisely said nothing until months later, when I went to visit him in England and we decided on a trip to Italy. It started with a sudden kiss as our plane touched down in Rome. A few days later, we were in a café in Sorrento, giddy with romance, going back and forth with that delighted conversation that goes, "I have a question for you, when did you first…" etc., when he asked, "I have a question for you, do you have any idea how much I love you?"

I was too flustered to say anything, so I just laughed. But I should have said no, Simon, actually I have no idea. Usually you never find out really, because usually you're never tested; you skate on the surface of an ordinary life, not realizing how lucky you are that the ice is holding you up.

By this point I'm trying to decide who the pallbearers should be. If there are usually six pallbearers and three spots are taken with my one brother and Simon's two brothers, that only leaves three more. If I choose a representative from groups of friends, say, friends from university, neighbors, and colleagues, would Casey be offended if I picked Paul? I don't want there to be any hard feelings. By now I am getting a bit stressed.

It doesn't help that when my writers' group reviews this chapter, Peter says, "What about me?" He is only partly joking. I'm completely dismayed. I can't believe I forgot about Peter. My buddy from book club, my date for plays at the Young People's Theatre from before I met Simon. I was the one who officiated at his Toronto Island wedding to Richard just a short while ago, for heaven's sake. I'm distraught about my oversight. I tell my friend Laura about it. "But what about Sigis?" is her only response, referring to her husband. I can't believe this.

When I tell Simon, he shrugs.

"Pallbearers should be the same height" is his only comment. I didn't know that, but it makes sense.

"Like how hard it was when we were portaging," I say.

Simon is more than a foot taller than I am, so it was really challenging to balance the canoe between us. He nods and adds, "Or at least they should be in pairs of the same height."

I decide to worry about the height of the pallbearers later. I'm more concerned with the question of how much lead time, exactly, I would need to book Patricia O'Callaghan. Simon and I once saw her perform at The Senator, a downtown jazz club. There were only a dozen or so people there. I was eating three feet from where she was singing and she literally brushed by me during the intermission. I stopped her to say how much I loved her music and she seemed genuinely appreciative. So how expensive and unavailable could she really be? But there's also the matter of booking the Canadian Children's Opera Company. I've got a cast of thousands now and what if they're not available?

It seems pretty heartless to call while Simon is still alive, but if I wait until after it might be too late. This is Toronto after all. If you want to go on a camping trip to any of the nearby provincial parks, you have to be on the Internet at exactly 7 a.m., five months before your planned weekend, to book a site. If you want to have friends over for dinner, you have to give them at least a month's notice and several alternative dates. And I want to get as much done as possible while I still have the energy and spirits to do so. It's at this point that I suddenly see myself from the outside, rather than the inside, where I usually live. I refrain from actually contacting anyone. After all, I don't want people to think I have a problem.

My friend Lisa says this is called "catastrophic thinking." You think that if you're prepared for a catastrophe, it will not happen. I think of it in terms of circumvention. Because the gods don't like it when your expectations are met, you trick them, by expecting something bad. This is as close as I come to having a religious belief system. My gods are plural, because I was born in India; and my hopes of them are modest, because I grew up in Canada.

Then, on April 28, 2014, while I was at Sunnybrook Hospital's emergency department for something minor, I was told I had leukemia. It was advanced, it was aggressive, and, if I did not start treatment immediately, it would kill me. Turns out the person I should have been worrying about was myself; the funeral I should have been planning was my own. Not that it's a total waste. I would be happy to use Simon's funeral arrangements for myself. It's just that I won't be there to enjoy them.

CHAPTER TWO

THE BEGINNING was a pain in the butt—literally. Hemorrhoids, of all things. To tell the truth, I did not even know what hemorrhoids were until I got them. I was just vaguely aware that they were something embarrassing that people laughed about. But I certainly was not laughing. I refer to my condition obliquely at work, as a "stomach ailment" or "lower back pain" ("Very low," Simon would add) that I am trying to get to "the bottom of." And I try to hide the related accoutrements: the doughnut-shaped pillow, the Epsom salts, the sitz bath, the ointments. My family doctor refers me to a clinic downtown for a surgical procedure that causes me more agonizing pain than I've ever felt before, and that doesn't even help in the end. I won't name the clinic or the doctor here because I don't want to get sued.

When the mad scientist doctor with the flyaway hair finishes torturing me, I sit gingerly across from him in his office, with my lips pressed tightly together, tears still streaking my face, while he writes me out a Percocet prescription for the pain. At first, I'm all like "I can't take Percocet!" I know how addictive it is. I even organized a panel at a law conference about Percocet. But when I experience the floating ease, the miraculous relief Percs bring, I go from being leery of them to scoping out my own independent sources. When my prescription runs out on a Sunday, the day before my follow-up appointment, I call every doctor friend I have to beg for a renewal.

My friend Homer, a trauma surgeon at Sunnybrook Hospital, who was not at home during my first desperate wave of messages, calls me back the next day, alarmed.

"I didn't get your message until today. I don't use that voice mail. Vivian heard it and said you sounded strange."

"It's okay," I reassure him dreamily, "I got the prescription, didn't mean to scare you. Don't worry."

"Look," he says, obviously worried, "there could be an internal infection. Let me check with a specialist I know, a prof at U. of T. I'll call you right back."

He calls again minutes later. "Yeah, he says you should really get a CT scan to check it out. Can you come to Sunnybrook emerg?"

"Right now?" I ask.

"Yeah, I can meet you there in half an hour."

I pause before I answer. I was feeling good by then, lying in bed, eating Cheetos, and rereading Jane Austen's *Persuasion* for approximately the millionth time. I had just reached the best part where Captain Wentworth pours out his soul to Anne in a letter:

Dare not say that man forgets sooner than woman, that his love has an earlier death. I have loved none but you. Unjust I may have been, weak and resentful I have been, but never inconstant.

However, Homer's tone, and especially his offer to meet me there, makes it sound a little urgent, so I sigh, "Fine," as if I'm the one doing him the favor.

I get up reluctantly and hide my snacks in my night table drawer so my eleven-year-old twins will not find them. I would give my life for the twins, but not my Cheetos. I call a cab because Sunnybrook is close to our house and parking there would cost more than the cab fare. The children are both out: Anna at a rehearsal with her opera chorus, and Jack at a guitar lesson. The kitchen is noisy with sizzling beef and our ancient clattering exhaust fan. Simon is in the middle of making lasagna for dinner, little suspecting that we are about to eat more lasagna in the next six months than we have eaten in our entire lives to date (on *Family Feud* it would register number one in "Top ten dishes people bring you in a crisis").

The emergency department has a ridiculous setup. Instead of asking you to take a number, a sign simply directs you to sit in the front row of chairs that face the nurses' triage rooms. People have to work out the order for themselves. After sitting there for a few hours, I see that the person at the beginning of the row goes up when the nurse calls out, "Who's next?" Then everyone shuffles over one seat.

Seeing as we're all there for something awful, the idea of eventually sitting in every single germy seat, one after the other, is disturbing. I mean, some people are moaning with pain, some are vomiting into basins, some are oddly swollen. Still, we just shuffle along, seat to seat. Because we're Canadian, when there are seats to spare, people do not sit directly beside someone, but leave exactly equidistant gaps (as we do on the subway), which means that as more people arrive and fill in the gaps, we are now out of order and have to remember who arrived first.

When the row fills up, people have to sit elsewhere in the waiting room and keep track a whole other way until they can claim a seat in the front row. Every single, solitary time someone new arrives, someone in the front row would explain the entire mysterious procedure all over again. Why can't they have one of those things that you use at the deli counter of a grocery store, you know what I mean? Where you rip off a little number?

I'm still wondering what the name of that thing is (I look it up later—turns out it's called a Take-a-Number dispenser, which I probably should have guessed), when I get my consultation with the triage nurse, routine blood work, and CT scan. While I'm lying on a bed in a little chamber off the emergency room to await the results, a young man in green scrubs, who is either a resident, medical intern, or high school student (he looks that young), rushes in and demands, "Have you lost a lot of blood recently?" I don't have the slightest idea what he means. I actually look down at my arms and legs in case I have injuries I have been unaware of and am gushing blood. I do not see anything untoward, so I answer tentatively, "I don't think so, no."

"Because you have almost no hemoglobin," he tells me. "You need a transfusion right away." I'm very confused. I'm notoriously unobservant (walking right by our house on my way home from work; not noticing Simon has set up an eight-foot-high Christmas tree in our living room until the children mention it at dinner), but surely even I could not have failed to notice losing copious amounts of blood? A nurse sets me up with an IV line for a blood transfusion minutes later, along with an infusion of pain medication, so I'm feeling drowsy and strangely relaxed, enjoying the fact I am tucked cozily under a heated flannel blanket, when Homer comes in and pulls up the wheeled stool by my bed.

He sits down, rests one hand on my knee, over the blanket that is no longer warm, and says quietly and evenly, "Your blood test results show you have leukemia."

My first thought is "No, they don't."

Because this is not how the "you-have-cancer" script goes. Surely he knows that. He is a doctor, for heaven's sake. He is supposed to say, "There might be something that needs to be checked out. It's probably nothing, but we need more tests to be sure." He would then book a series of tests for me. Then weeks would go by and eventually I would be diagnosed. I even voice part of that script by asking, "Don't you need to do more tests to confirm?"

"No," he says, without hesitating.

"It's definite, the blasts are everywhere. You need to be admitted tonight." He also says, "You're going to be okay. In two years, you'll look back on this as just something that happened."

He means it as reassuring, but the words explode in my ears. I skip right over his "You're going to be okay" because I cannot even register the possibility of being anything other than okay. What I register are the words "two years." Two. Years. I cannot fathom being sick for that long. It is incomprehensible. I barely even get colds. I take on average two or three sick days a year. I've never smoked a cigarette in my life, much less tried any illegal drugs. I don't drink alcohol. I love to swim, canoe, hike. I can't have cancer. I can't be sick for two years.

Homer calls Simon. Simon calls our neighbors first, Marta and Pierre, to stay with Jack and Anna, and then he calls my parents. Soon everyone is at the hospital with me. There is nowhere private to talk. I have been moved to the hallway at this point, waiting for a bed in the cancer ward to become available. My mother tears off bits of a slice of cheese pizza she managed to get from somewhere and feeds it to me while we meet with the hematologist who will be in charge of my treatment.

He tells me that I have acute myeloid leukemia, which will kill me if left untreated. The treatment will be one round of induction chemotherapy in hospital and then two rounds of consolidation chemo as an outpatient. The first round will take one week to administer, but I will have to remain in hospital for three more weeks to recover from it. The next two rounds will similarly take a week each, with three weeks to recover each time, but I can do those treatments from home. I will then need three months to recover from the treatment as a whole. I will be back at work in six months, November 1, 2014. The hallway is so brightly lit and noisy with passing people you would never know this conversation is happening after midnight. And even though it is so late, Homer remains there in the passageway with us.

Homer and I have known each other since grade 7, and we started dating in grade 11, when he was fifteen and I was sixteen (he had skipped a grade). He has always had a special place in my heart as the first boy I ever loved. We were top students, luckily in a school where that did not make you a social outcast. At a grade 12 year-end assembly, where joke awards were passed out, the band teacher and strings teacher, whom everyone suspected were having an affair, got the Couple That Plays Together Stays Together Award, while we got the Wholesome Couple of the Year Award (a loaf of whole wheat bread).

Homer was addicted to the TV show *M*A*S*H* and his ambition was to be an army surgeon like Hawkeye Pierce. He became exactly that, ultimately joining the Canadian Armed Forces to pay his way through medical school and then enduring several tours of duty operating on injured soldiers in Kandahar, Afghanistan. I wanted to be a writer and it took me a lot longer, but I guess I ended up being that as well. Our relationship ended when we graduated from high school and went on to different universities, but our friendship never did. It was my idea for him to intersperse his essay for his medical school application with lines from the John Donne poem that begins "No man is an island." I thought the ending so perfectly described what I always thought of as his unselfish (but which I dismissed in other lesser people as self-aggrandizing) desire to be a doctor: "And therefore, never send to know for whom the bell tolls; It tolls for thee." I believed in literature the way he believed in science.

We had both come to Canada as very young children—he from Taiwan, I from India—with parents who did not end up working in jobs commensurate with their abilities. I always felt bad about my parents' thwarted ambitions—the biochemistry lab my mother should have been running, the metallurgical engineering my father should have been studying. Homer, though, was not given to pity, not for himself, and not for others. When asked to do something around the house, he would mock his father, "You have a PhD, you open the jar."

Our parents believed in education above all else. When I was in my early twenties I had all four wisdom teeth removed one morning and fainted that evening at the dinner table. I groggily regained consciousness to find a firefighter in full gear looming over me asking me questions I could hear, but did not have the breath to answer.

"Does she speak English?" he asked my mother, who had been hovering worriedly nearby in our cramped kitchen.

She drew herself up, completely offended. "She went to *Stanford*," my mother informed him, which to an Indian parent is a more pertinent piece of information for a medic than a blood type. If there had been room, I'm sure she would have insisted that fact be engraved, along with my grade point average, on the MedicAlert bracelet I now wear.

All through my childhood my mother foisted upon me biographies of famous people: Thomas Edison, Marie Curie, Charles Dickens, hoping to inspire me, I guess. But all I gleaned from them was the suspicion that I could not be destined for greatness because I had never suffered, never worked in a blacking warehouse at the age of eleven, pasting labels on bottles like Dickens had. I would tell my mother accusingly that I would never be famous and it was all her fault because my childhood was too happy.

For Homer and me, a fun afternoon in high school meant taking a long walk from our suburban subdivisions all the way to Rosedale, where Toronto's old money lives, and picking out the mansion that would one day be ours. I would peruse catalogs of foster children to sponsor (just pennies a day!) from those international aid organizations, thinking we could start there, and then when we grew up, move on to adopting actual children plucked from the streets of China and India. We were going to save lives, literally and figuratively, with our scalpels and our pens and our sheer belief in ourselves and each other. We were going to rule the world and save it at the same time. So really it is not bizarrely coincidental at all, but rather poetically just, that when the bell tolled, I did not have to send to know anything, Homer was there to tell me.

CHAPTER THREE

A PERSON'S RESPONSE to hearing they have a life-threatening illness is apparently similar to their response to the death of a loved one—namely, grief. There are either five or seven stages of grief, depending on your Google searches. The typical five are denial, anger, bargaining, depression, and acceptance. If you go for seven, the experts throw in shock and guilt, in no particular order. I don't know how long each stage lasts—in one of my favorite *Simpsons* episodes, Homer Simpson goes through all of them in 10 seconds—but I know I am in denial for a very long time.

I start with the firm belief that being confined to hospital for a month is something I can make the best of by making it as pleasant as possible for myself. Instead of learning more about my diagnosis or getting second opinions about treatment options, the first thing I want is for Simon to set up a visiting schedule for me.

"What kind of time slots do you want?" he asks.

I propose every half hour, starting at 9 a.m. and ending at 8 p.m., with an hour off for lunch and an hour off for dinner.

"Don't you want time to rest?"

"Oh no," I say airily. "But I think you should limit it to two people per half hour, I don't want more than that." I feel I am showing a lot of restraint.

My first full day in hospital I have eleven visitors, not counting Simon and my mother. It was a good thing Simon had brought in two folding chairs from home (the hospital supplied only one bedside armchair). People bring me chocolate and fruit and flowers, and even my next month's book club selection conveniently downloaded onto an iPod.

Homer, who looks in on me often, disapproves of my having anyone other than family visit, because of the infection risk. "But my doctor said it was good to have visitors!" I tell him. "He said studies show people who have visitors do *better* than people who don't."

He presses his lips together. "Are they randomized studies?" he demands. "Did they take a million patients and then randomly assign visitors to some and no visitors to others?

"Of course not," he goes on, answering his own question. "No one could ethically do a study like that. So you can't say visitors help, and we do know they can spread infection."

I see my doctor soon afterwards, but I don't get a chance to ask him again about my number of visitors. He is there to soberly explain what he has discovered about my particular genetic mutation. Of course it is during dinner (one of the few hospital dinners I can actually tolerate), cheese ravioli with tomato sauce that gradually grows cold and congeals as I struggle to follow his explanation, more concerned about my dinner than my DNA.

He explains that my cancer cells are caused specifically by pieces of chromosome 4 peeling off and exchanging places with chromosome 11, and chromosome 7 exchanging places with chromosome 10. That's causing the mutations (also called "blasts"), which are the leukemia cells, and it's associated with a more difficult to treat leukemia. I picture a kind of morbid square dance where partners peel off and join other partners they're not supposed to join, while the fiddler, my body's immune system, looks the other way and fiddles on obliviously. My doctor says they don't know why cells start doing this, they have yet to link it to any known cause. It does not appear to be environmental or genetic. It's referred to as "idiopathic," I guess because that sounds better than shrugging your shoulders and saying "Search me."

It is possible, and indeed quite probable, that the above paragraph is a wildly inaccurate summary of what my doctor told me that evening. He is a brilliant and highly respected hematologist (he went to Harvard, according to my mother, who looked up his credentials). But what I'm doing is what I will continue to do throughout these pages: I'm relaying what I heard, and even though it is based on notes I jotted down in my journal at the time, it still may be very different from what was said. My scientific background ends with grade 12 chemistry; and while I did google stages of grief, and while I would later google Dante's circles of hell (expecting to find one of them is a cancer ward), I never once googled leukemia, or cancer, or treatments for same.

My only question at the time, which I don't voice, is why

tell me things I cannot control? Is knowledge power or is ignorance bliss? I seriously toy with putting in a request to be told nothing, on the grounds that it will only upset me, even though that goes against everything we hold sacred in this information age. Isn't it better, I fret, to be happily ignorant and eat my dinner in peace? Wouldn't that be better for my health than to have my stomach clench with worry and fear and leave my ravioli uneaten? I never do make that request, but I ignore the "what," the hard facts, even as my friend Kate is searching the Internet night and day, basically going to medical school on my behalf. Instead, I spend my time on the "why," trying to relate to my cancer cells on a personal level, trying to understand what makes them tick.

I would add an eighth stage to the stages of grief: betrayal. All this time, I had thought of my mind and body as being on the same team. And now I feel like my body wants to kill me, and I feel betrayed. I try asking Homer why my cells are doing this.

"Don't they realize that if I die, they die too? Aren't they motivated by self-interest to survive at least? What's the point of killing their host? They need me. Don't we have bacteria that live in us all the time? Why can't cancer cells do that? Isn't it in their best interests to keep me alive? Don't they want to live?"

"You know, they don't actually have emotions," Homer answers, patiently explaining, without a hint of derision in his voice (which is pretty impressive, considering the nonsense I'm spouting) that there is no point inquiring too closely into what motivates a chromosome.

I find that hard to believe because I ascribe emotions to

everything. I know, for instance, that my house loves me, that my small leather knapsack is loyal, and that my computer thinks I'm an idiot. Even the hair on my head I consider as having aspirations that are separate and apart from my own. Some of my hair manages to survive the first round of chemo, and I admire its tenacity. Way to go, I think. Way to cling to life even in the face of such an assault.

I thought I would lose all my hair immediately because that's the classic image I have of a cancer patient, completely bald. But it actually takes a long time because I have a lot of hair. Every day I rake through it with my fingers and come away with clumps and clumps.

"Do you want a bag to keep it in? As a memento?" asks one of the nurses sentimentally when she spies an entire nest of it on my bed.

"Ick, no" is my unsentimental and revolted response.

When I tell Simon about it, he says he's been meaning to ask me if I would like him to shave his head in solidarity. I look at him in disbelief and blurt, "Are you insane?" before belatedly adding, "But that's nice of you, to offer, I mean... uh, thanks."

A few months before, at a party, I had run into a lawyer I know who had been battling cancer herself. When I exclaimed about how good she looked, she instantly whipped out her cellphone to show me photos of when she was completely bald. Meanwhile, since my hair really started to go, I haven't looked at myself in the mirror without my cap on. I have no idea what my head looks like right now, much less have photographic evidence of it. It was a friend who sent me the cap, a beautiful coral pink, streaked with silver, that ties on easily with a bow to one side. (Think cancer patient meets 1920s flapper.)

My first hospital roommate is going through the same hair loss at the same time as I am. It turns out she and her husband own the Halloween supply store that Simon and I take Jack and Anna to every year to buy accessories for their costumes.

"She said she's planning to use Halloween wigs from their store," I tell him.

"Which ones?" he asks with interest. And we run through the ones we remember: sexy nurse, vampire vixen, bride of Frankenstein.

Jack and Anna are unperturbed by my baldness.

"Terry Fox's hair came back in curly!" Anna informs me cheerfully during one visit. "It used to be straight before."

"Cool," I say, "I always used to wish I had curly hair." Neither of us mentions that Terry Fox did not make it.

I had started chemo on May 1, three days after my admission to the cancer ward, but the first few days didn't seem terrible at all. I'm not nauseous; I'm not especially tired; I can chat with friends who visit. I bask in compliments about how brave I am. I nobly announce that really, I've had it so good until now that even if I were the one responsible for handing out cancer (and I can picture that as an actual job, albeit not a very popular one) I'd be, if not the first, definitely one of the first people I'd give it to. Like it's my turn for a tragedy. Like it's only fair.

"This isn't so bad!" I tell Homer proudly, when he drops by midway through the chemo. But he doesn't echo my enthusiasm. "You're in a marathon," he warns me. "You're not even a quarter way through yet." I pout, annoyed with him for raining on my parade, for stopping me from using denial as a shortcut to bravery. But he is right. The chemo hits me toward the end of the seven-day course, because it's the cumulative effect of the drugs that knocks you out, not the daily infusions.

Chemo works by killing rapidly dividing cells, which include, of course, the cancer cells that are the target of the drug, but also all other rapidly dividing cells—your infection-fighting T-cells, which are found in your blood and in a particular bend of your bowel (which is why you become prone to digestive problems such as diarrhea and worse), your hair cells, which is why you lose your hair, and even your taste buds, which is why you lose your appetite.

Once the effects of the chemo hit me, I suddenly do not want visitors and we abruptly suspend my crazy visiting schedule. But even though I cancel visits from friends, there is still an endless stream of official people who come to call when you're in the hospital: student volunteers who offer to help you do simple movement exercises; older volunteers with carts of magazines and books; nursing managers who want to know if you're satisfied with the nursing services you're receiving; and nutritionists who push samples of high-protein powders on you to up your calorie count and leave charts where you are to tick off your food preferences in great detail, right down to the number of packets of sugar you want with your tea.

Also, I agree whenever I'm asked to participate in a research project, and that means giving extra vials of blood, and being interviewed almost daily about responses to blood transfusions.

I'm in the control group that did not get the irradiated blood, though I don't think I was supposed to know that.

I reach my limit, though, with the minister who keeps dropping by (while there may be no atheists in the trenches, there still are atheists in the cancer wards), because he always comes accompanied by two women whose job descriptions I forget. While it might be possible for someone who is despairing to reach out and bare their soul to a single kindly person, religious or not, I can't believe that anyone would feel comfortable baring their soul to a bureaucratic committee of three. It's a pointless exercise, and I put in a request for them not to visit, which they eventually respect.

The most disconcertingly named regular visitors are members of the "pain and palliative care team." I think they're doctors, but I'm not sure. Their job is to monitor my level of pain and my dosages of pain medication. The first time they visit, I'm so alarmed by their name I ask about it, because it makes it seem like I'm dying if I need "palliative care." One of the team members explains that to "palliate" just means to "alleviate" pain, so it is an entirely appropriate name. It's as if she's on a mission to rehabilitate the term. I'm not convinced, and much later, at home, I look up the word in my *Canadian Oxford Dictionary*. It defines "palliative" as "anything used to alleviate pain, anxiety, etc. especially without eliminating its source." However, it defines "palliative care" as "medical care provided for the terminally ill, aimed at relieving symptoms." So I consider that I'm right after all. And they really do need to change their name.

I'm full of other helpful suggestions as well. When a surgical resident installs my Hickman line—a thin, flexible tube he inserts into the large vein above my heart for delivering chemotherapy and blood products, and for taking blood for tests—I'm upset, because he doesn't speak to me at all. Not one word. I don't know what he's doing, and I don't even know when he's finished until he abruptly leaves the room. He has the accent of a villain in a James Bond movie. I complain about it to my medical team (not the accent, but the fact he didn't say anything to me) and they listen sympathetically.

"Even though it didn't hurt, it was worse than that thing that did hurt…" I pause, trying to remember the name of that earlier procedure. "The bone marrow biopsy!"

The biopsy was one of the first things they did, inserting a long needle deep into my hip to extract liquid from my bone marrow to see what percentage of the sample was cancer cells. A resident did it, under supervision of my doctor. Or rather, she tried to do it. After two attempts, the doctor took over. It was the first time I heard the dreaded phrase "You may feel a little pressure." It hurt, a lot, but the doctor was so kind and supportive, complimenting us both on what a great job we were doing, that I came out of it feeling good, even though the resident's part was unsuccessful and my part consisted of trying to keep my moaning to a minimum.

My medical team listens attentively. They think this is a good example of how bedside manner is as important as technical proficiency. And I feel proud to think that my experience matters, like I've contributed something to the issue of patient care.

There is one pain doctor I adore, because he explains things so well. I'm very surprised to hear from him that they have the ability to manage pain so well that no medical procedure should be painful (more for that hemorrhoid clinic to answer for!). He also says you should not be a martyr and wait for the pain to be unbearable before seeking relief, because then you are always playing catch-up. You have to get on top of it and take the medication before the pain is at its worst, so that you can battle it before it gets out of control. Since I was never one with remotely martyr-like tendencies, this all makes perfect sense to me.

I hit a snag, though, in my ability to control when I get the pills. When I feel the pain starting, I page the nurse, but it takes time for someone to answer the page, and then varying amounts of time for the paged nurse to get the pain pills. This is entirely understandable as I'm not the only patient, and I can see the nurses are run off their feet. So then I start to ask for the pills before I actually need them, my plan being to hoard them until I do need them. That way, I can wait for the exact right moment to take the pills, not too soon, not too late. For a while, that plan works. But then the night shift is taken over by a brisk young nurse I haven't had before, pretty and pink-cheeked, in bright pink scrubs. But all that pinkness and youth is deceiving, to say the least. She is the toughest of all the nurses.

The first time she hands me the pills in a tiny medicine cup, I thank her politely and place the cup carefully on my bedside tray for later. She narrows her eyes.

"I have to see you take them."

"Why?" I stall.

"Because they're a narcotic and that's the rule with narcotics. I'd get into serious trouble otherwise. I have to make a note of the time you ingest them."

She never comes right out and says so, but I infer that the issue is that a patient could stockpile the little pills and then commit suicide through overdose. And Simon thinks they're also worried I might sell the pills, which I couldn't really imagine happening from a hospital bed, but I guess others are more entrepreneurial than I am.

"I can be trusted!" I tell her, laughing in what I hope is an entirely trustworthy and non-suicidal way.

She doesn't smile, but stands there waiting for me to swallow the pills, which I meekly do, after a brief mental struggle about which would be better—to take the pills when I don't yet actually need them, or to admit I had wasted her time and called for them too early. I go with the former because I think getting a girl-who-cried-wolf reputation would hurt me more than taking unnecessary pills just this one time.

I appeal to one of the doctors on my team the next time he does his rounds. "Can't you write that on my chart? That they can give me the pills without watching me take them, and then I can take them when I need them?"

"No," he says, "those are the rules.

"But," he adds helpfully, "you could pretend to take them and then you'll have them for later."

Unorthodox and surprising though his advice is, I do think about it seriously, but end up dismissing it. The pills are the powdery kind, not the smooth gel kind. If I put them in my mouth, they would start to dissolve immediately, so I couldn't spit them out later once the nurse left. On the other hand, if I try to fake-take them, and drop them instead, I'm afraid I would lose the tiny white pills in my white sheets. Then I wouldn't have them, but they would be marked as having been taken, which would mean I would have to wait the required three hours before my next allowed dose, which would be worse than taking them early. So, as much as I appreciate his trying to help me, I do nothing except fume at the nurse.

Then comes the night I think I'm dying. It is not a dream or hallucination. It is much too real for that. It feels like it's happening. I'm rushing through the universe at a terrifying rate. I have never before felt the sensation of traveling so fast, faster than the screaming downturn of any roller coaster, so fast that the points of light of the stars surrounding me are blurring into blazing multicolored streams and I have no control over the force and the terror and the speed. I am sure this is it, and it is all too fast to even take a breath or cry out or feel anything other than fear at the heart-stopping speed. Then I open my eyes and I am in bed, gasping and sobbing.

She's there. Her pink scrubs glow even in the darkness. She puts her arms around my shoulders and says, "You are not alone."

CHAPTER FOUR

MAKE THE BEEPING STOP, I want to wail and tear out the little hair I have left. But it never stops. When air bubbles are trapped in my Hickman line, my IV pump starts a pattern—*beep beep BEEP beep*—that it repeats over and over. It happens a dozen times a day and is multiplied by all the patients, in all the rooms, in all the ward. If ignored, the beeps get louder and *louder* and *LOUDER*. And the pump's beeping is often ignored because, apparently, its needs are not as urgent as its jangling cry suggests.

I press my call button. "…help you?" crackles the voice on the intercom high on the wall above my bed.

"My IV is beeping," I call out.

"What?" She can't hear me above the beeping.

My mother leaps up. "Her IV! It's beeping!"

The intercom switches off. Then I hear the page, "Nurse to room 43C, nurse to room 43C." A nurse eventually whizzes in and turns off the alarm by pressing a button. She scrutinizes the lines, flicks at the air bubbles several times, then restarts the pump. Seconds after she leaves, it starts beeping again.

Sometimes, in my chemo-induced fog, I cannot tell if it is my pump, or my roommate's. I try to listen as closely as I can. I reach out shakily, trying to turn the stand to face me so I can see if the lights are also flashing, which will let me know if it is my pump. Often it's my roommate's, but she's sleeping through it. So I press the call button and try to explain it is the next bed, not my own. I feel it's important to make this distinction in case someone, somewhere, is keeping track of who presses their call buttons the most, who are the most troublesome patients. I don't want this call in *my* column. I worry when, despite my explanation through the intercom, it's my nurse they send in instead of my neighbor's nurse.

"It's actually her IV, not mine," I say apologetically, pointing at the curtain. Drat, for sure this is going to go in my column now.

I lucked out with my room assignment, even though it contains three patients, instead of the more typical two, because I am the farthest one from the door, so I have the most privacy and more windows. No one has to walk by me to get to the other patients. My narrow hospital bed touches the wall at my head. To my right is a curtain separating me from the middle bed. You can stand between my bed and the curtain, but you would be touching both if you did so. To my left is a window that runs the length of the wall, with a nice wide sill to put stuff on. But you have to be careful not to block the air vents as it is boiling hot on the ward. There is room for a chair between the windowsill and my bed. But in order to sit in the chair, you would have to climb over it first, as there is no room to walk by it.

At the foot of my bed are two closets (even though only one is mine, I commandeer both to store my folding chairs), and another window that runs the length of the room. There's a control pad on one side of my bed, and although it always takes me several contortions, often jackknifing me in the middle as both the head and foot of the bed rise up, I eventually manage to raise the bed as high as it will go. Almost every morning I have the same conversation.

"Why is this bed so high?" The nurse will frown as she reaches to press the button that lowers it. "You could fall."

"No, don't—" I put out my hand to stop her. "The view," I say. "I want to see the trees." It's May and they are just starting to bud.

An eighty-five-year-old old woman is in the worst bed, by the door; worst because she gets the noise and light from the hall and she is right beside the bathroom. She is the perfect roommate because she sleeps all day and has no visitors. She is not being treated for cancer. She is waiting for a nursing home spot to open up. It seems like a crazy waste of a precious cancer bed with its 24/7 top-notch medical and nursing care. She can walk, but refuses everybody's attempts to get her up. She can use the bathroom, but chooses to go in diapers instead. (I hear the nurses complaining about that.) Except for one scare in the night when they thought she was having a stroke or something, it's like there's no one in that bed at all.

In the middle bed is a woman in her sixties getting dialysis; she has replaced the woman who owns the Halloween store. She speaks only a little English, but she is always trying to chat with me or offer me help in some way. She has millions of family visitors and when they're not there she speaks on her phone nonstop. But luckily she and her visitors all speak quietly, and in some musical language I don't recognize, so it feels like a murmur of background noise to me. If it were an unending conversation I could actually follow, it would drive me mad.

I don't have the energy to talk on the phone or even watch Netflix. I just stare out the window at the trees, or at the flowers, sent by friends, that line my corner of the room. There's a cluster of striped tulips on my left beside a curving white orchid. And there's an elaborate arrangement on the windowsill at the foot of my bed: deep red roses, blushing lilies, each perfectly placed, down to the last leaf. But, one morning, I notice they look different. I've been gazing at them so long I can tell that the flowers are slightly askew. I'm confused at first, but then, through half-closed eyes, I catch my roommate shuffling over to refresh the water. She yanks them up, pours in some water she's carried from the bathroom in a Styrofoam cup, and plunks them back in. I'm distressed.

"Do you think it would be okay if I ask her, you know, *nicely,* and everything, not to touch them?" I fret to Simon.

He doesn't answer my question, and instead asks, "Did you notice what flowers she has?"

"No."

"Take a look," he advises me.

Next time I go to the bathroom, I discreetly glance over at her bed. On her bedside table is a tiny vase with a single rose; it is artificial.

I don't say anything to her about my flowers.

After I complete the week of chemo, I keep getting fevers. My mother works nonstop putting cold compresses on my head and legs to bring the fevers down. When she leaves for the night, I continue to do it myself. I struggle a bit and my neighbor hears me. She hurries over and starts wringing out the washcloths and places them on my legs herself. I weakly try to tell her to stop.

"You're being too kind," I say. "You're sick yourself. Don't worry about me."

When she returns to her bed, I suddenly have a less grateful, more alarmed, thought. Wait a minute, she is sick herself! I'm not even having healthy people visit right now—I can't be having sick people touch me! I panic and, instead of waiting to ask the doctor about it, I tell my mother when she arrives the next day. She immediately asks the nurse to tell that patient she should not be touching me.

That evening, when my neighbor's family arrives, they suddenly start conversing in an agitated manner rather than in their usual soft tones. So even though I cannot understand a word, I feel sure they are offended and are talking about me. I want desperately to apologize for giving offense and to explain that I was just worried because I have no immune system, but I don't have the breath to do it.

Luckily she is so sweet that she still acts the same toward me. And, as I gain strength, I chat more with her and worry less about her infecting me. One day she lends me a fashion magazine, which I leaf through out of politeness, even though I am not particularly interested, pleased with myself that I am now being a friendly roommate. Of course, five seconds after I return the magazine, her nurse whisks the curtains closed around her, puts up a hazard sign, and sets up a toilet by her bed. It turns out she's being isolated because she has an infection, and I worry that I have put my life at risk, merely to be polite.

In the meantime, the old woman at the far end finally gets her nursing home spot, only to be replaced by a woman in her late forties who radiates hostility like waves of heat you can actually feel. She complains about everything at the top of her voice: the noise in the room, the terrible nurses, the useless workmen who are renovating her home, her father who doesn't visit.

I'm terrified of her.

"I've never even made eye contact with her," I confide to Simon.

"I did," Simon reports. "I even said hello."

I'm impressed. "What did she say?"

"She just scowled."

I try never to look at her when I get up to use the bathroom. My practice had been to almost close the door when leaving, but not to click it shut because the old woman was always sleeping and I thought the loud click would wake her. But when I do it this time, as I shuffle away from the bathroom, I hear hostile woman get up in a huff and ostentatiously click the door shut. The next time I use the bathroom, there is a little handwritten sign taped to it (in capital letters) saying, PLEASE SHUT THE BATHROOM DOOR COMPLETELY!

She leaves, after about a week, on a day I am feeling well, so I am sitting in a chair instead of my bed and from that vantage point I can see my neighbor and her daughter, who is visiting. I point to the empty far bed and say, "I'm so glad she's gone!"

That unleashes a fervent rush of agreement from the woman and even from her daughter, who says, "I know, right?" And we have a lot of fun talking about how mean that woman was. I feel that it heals the rift I had been sensing between my neighbor's family and myself, because there is nothing that brings two people together more than complaining about a third.

Now that we've bonded, I'm shocked one day to hear a nurse, through the curtain, reminding her loudly and matter-of-factly that she only has six months to live. It seems a strange thing for the nurse to do. Surely you would remember such news? Yet Simon and I sit there picking at our sandwiches on the other side of the curtain, listening to the nurse saying, "You know your prognosis is six months, right?"

The woman murmurs something. Then the nurse continues in the same forthright tone, "And you know, if you stop the dialysis, it will be a peaceful way to die."

CHAPTER FIVE

THERE IS A PROBLEM with the Internet connection in my room. It was there at first and then it was gone. Simon takes my laptop and says he'll try to find a connection elsewhere. The cleaning woman comes in as he's preparing to leave. We usually chat a bit when she arrives. I've learned, for instance, that she's originally from Poland and that she's been working at Sunnybrook for more than ten years. But this time, before saying anything, she efficiently sweeps all around my bed, making a pile of my hair and the tops of syringes the nurses use to flush my IV lines.

"Your husband," she then says abruptly, tilting her head at Simon's departing back, "I watch. He don't leave."

She nods at me. I am about to say he did leave, but only to check something, when it hits me what she means. My husband, he didn't leave me. He stayed. Unspoken is that not everyone sticks around a cancer ward.

Simon comes every single morning and sometimes again in the evening with Jack and Anna. He's a stay-at-home dad and has been ever since I returned to work after my maternity leave. Even while I'm in the hospital, he keeps their routine steady: homework, piano, board games or TV, bed. He does everything and acts like it's nothing. "Kate says you're too modest," I relayed to him once.

"I have so much to be modest about" was his quick response.

When Simon returns, he sighs as he sits down in the chair and slides the computer with a thump onto the windowsill.

"I can get a connection in the visitors' room outside the ward doors," he reports.

"Past the elevators?" I ask. "Not the visitors' room next door?"

"Not the one next door," he confirms.

"I think the food court works too," he adds. The food court is a few floors down, but it might as well be a world away. I can't imagine being around regular people, lining up, and buying and eating wraps and pizza and falafel, the cacophonous bustle, the competing smells.

He's trying to get me reconnected so I can read the responses to my first entry on CaringBridge. Kate set up the account for me. It's a free website meant to help sick people keep in touch with family and friends during an illness, or "health journey" as they so brightly put it. Rather than labor at trying to email all my friends individually, the idea is that I can post one entry that everyone (who has been given the password) can read. People can then post comments back. Simon has been posting brief entries from home, keeping friends up to date about how my treatment is going until I have the energy to do it myself.

Kate and I met in our first year of law school at the University of Toronto, and she has been there for every important milestone in my life. She spoke at my wedding and at my swearing-in as a judge. I joked then that her next speech would be the eulogy at my funeral, which is not so funny now. She ended her wedding speech for me by referring to one struggle we had shared, our sometimes despairing search for true love.

She described a single friend of hers who was fond of saying "Whenever another friend of mine gets married, a little piece of me dies," but said that she felt exactly the opposite; she felt the story of Simon and me finding each other in Africa is proof that "there really is a fairy tale waiting to be written for every one of us—we just have to get out our pens and start writing."

I am eventually able to release a small grateful post thanking everyone for the wave of support that lifted Simon, Jack, Anna, and me up before we even had the chance to sink under the weight of my diagnosis. Friends put up a meal schedule through the same website and it seems like every single person I have ever known is dropping off a dinner at our house: old friends, new friends, parents of Jack and Anna's friends, even classmates from law school I haven't seen in almost twenty years. Simon brings in leftovers to share with me: Vietnamese rice paper rolls, Mexican empanadas. When I ask who brought a particular dinner, he sometimes has no idea, he hadn't recognized the name at all.

Anna is perplexed. "Who are these people?" she would ask, as yet another person knocked at the door bearing a chicken pot pie. Very soon Simon's mother Tricia arrives from England to help Simon in any way she can, keeping the house clean, walking Anna to school, playing endless games of Scrabble with Jack, trying to keep things normal.

I am now impatiently waiting to see what the responses to my post are but am thwarted at every turn. Simon suggests asking one of the computer-savvy nurses for help, but he is not on duty that day. There is also the young orderly who had helped us the first time, but when we appeal to him now he doesn't know why the connection is no longer working when it had worked so easily at first.

He can't stay long to help us as he's on his rounds delivering large Styrofoam cups of ice water to every patient. I accept one from him even though I have scarcely touched my morning cup. I hoard them when he comes by, ever since my mother notified me in appalled accents that the nurse who delivers the water when he's not there fills a plastic bucket with water and ice and then dips the cups in along with her fingers, whereas he fills each cup individually, at the ice station.

In the end, I manage to connect with my office IT person for help. It's great, and not only because he's able to tell me how to change my computer's configurations to connect to the hospital's Internet provider, but because he refers to me respectfully as "Your Honor" whenever he tells me what to type next. The title, and even more than the title, the deference in his voice, is a surprise to me. Even though I've been in hospital for only a week, I'd already forgotten I was anything other than a sick person, or that I'd ever been anything other than a sick person.

Although the doctors and nurses and other staff are always extremely kind, there is a power imbalance as there always is between the strong and the weak, the adult and the child, the well and the sick. Suddenly I'm reminded I'm more than just a sick person. And, after days of trying, I now have bedside Internet access.

It seems counterintuitive that writing about being sick could serve as a distraction from being sick, but it's true. Author Dave Eggers writes that sharing pain dilutes it, and I agree. Lying awake in that dead zone between when they wake me up to take my vitals at 6:00 a.m. and when breakfast arrives at 8:00 a.m., I occupy myself by composing a post. In the background I hear a nurse speak sharply to someone in the visitors' room next door: "You're not allowed in here overnight!" People are always doing it, though; not everyone lives within a convenient drive of midtown Toronto, and not everyone can afford a hotel. I miss what the person says in response as I'm busy propping myself up with pillows. The concentration required intensifies my nausea, and my vision is a bit blurry, so I can't type very long. But although the typing is a chore, the composing is fun.

I lie awake and plan out my post in my head. I obsess over it until it's a relief to finally post it, because then I can stop thinking about it. It's like Dumbledore's Pensieve, the silver basin in which he places his thoughts when his head gets too full, so he can relax and examine them at his leisure later.

Really everything makes me think of Harry Potter because I practically know the books off by heart. I have read them out loud to Jack and Anna three full times (all seven volumes) and I was halfway through a fourth reading when I got sick. I have perfected my voices—I do an especially good Umbridge and Moaning Myrtle—and I now know better than to interrupt my reading to start a discussion. In the beginning, I often got sidetracked. When Harry gazed into the Mirror of Erised (which shows your heart's desire), I paused to ask Jack and Anna what they thought such a mirror would show them if they looked into it. Jack was having none of it.

"It would show *you*," he said promptly, "reading Harry Potter. Keep reading!"

CaringBridge is that mirror as well as that Pensieve. It shows both my hidden fears and my heart's desires. It sometimes looks like Jack's grade 2 journal. He took it very seriously and wrote down every single thing he did. I tried gently to suggest that, in years to come, when he looked back and read it, he would be more interested in what he was thinking about, rather than what he was doing. But he ignored my suggestion (as usual) and kept up with his almost-in-real-time entries. I remember one entry began, "Now I am walking down the stairs to the kitchen…" His teacher had to institute a three-page-a-week limit because of Jack and his minutely detailed, endless entries. He didn't realize it was because of him, and he came home one day and innocently told us that his teacher had announced she would just stop reading at three pages, no matter how much else they wrote.

I will try not to inflict so much detail on my own readers, but just like Jack's teacher, you are free to stop reading at any point.

CHAPTER SIX

MY MOTHER comes every morning and brings me breakfast, often French toast, kept warm in a Thermos, with a carefully wrapped bottle of maple syrup to accompany it. Sometimes that ends up being a problem. I was once happily halfway through my first slice when a nurse walked in and stopped in dismay.

"You're not supposed to eat anything before your scan this morning!"

"No one told me," I protested.

She checked my chart. "They sent an order in cancelling your breakfast tray."

But of course I mostly ignore the trays the hospital provides, so I did not notice that. She checked with the technician doing the test and luckily it turned out half a piece of French toast wasn't going to affect the test and it could still go ahead. The tests are endless and awful. Sometimes I have to have an empty stomach, sometimes I have to force myself to drink a disgusting two liters of something that smells like chlorine, and sometimes they hook me to an IV line that injects me with dye to provide contrast when they look at the results.

My mother usually stays until Simon arrives around 10 a.m. She comes back around 5 p.m. and brings me dinner. It's the Maharashtran food I crave: lentils and potato patties with tamarind sauce, crêpes made of chickpea flour and green onions, and my favorite dish made of tapioca (but savory, not sweet) that's cooked with a bit of oil, potatoes, ground peanuts, and fresh coriander and that you eat with yogurt. It's May, which means mango season, so she brings a couple every day, which she cuts up on the windowsill and gives to me in a literal, rather than the usually symbolic, offering of devotion. They're special Alphonso mangos from India, available in Indian grocery stores here in the spring. Originally cultivated by Portuguese settlers, they are deeply orange with perfect smooth flesh, not stringy like those big red mangos you more commonly see.

Simon has lunch with me every day, but rarely without interruptions.

"It's time for your rectal exam," a doctor says in the middle of one lunch.

"Can it wait until I finish my ice cream?" I ask.

"No problem."

"Thanks."

"Well," Simon says, at the thought of a dining establishment that insists on offering such services between courses, "I certainly won't be coming *here* again."

I'm doing so well with respect to eating that I actually

worry I will be the only cancer patient in history not to lose any weight. Then the full force of the chemo hits me. I get terrible diarrhea. I spend forty-five minutes in the bathroom, return weakly to my bed, only to turn around instantly, dragging my IV stand, to head right back to the bathroom. At first the doctors suspect I have *C. difficile*, a highly contagious, potentially life-threatening, intestinal infection. So I'm put in isolation with a special sign by my bed and I'm not allowed to use the communal bathroom. When Simon and my mother come to visit, they have to wear a hospital gown, mask, and gloves. A nurse sets up a makeshift toilet for me that is a wheelchair with a bedpan built into the seat. It sits inches from my food tray.

Eventually they confirm I don't have *C. difficile* and the isolation is ended. I still don't feel like eating. Simon tries to insist. His formerly gentle tone becomes steely.

"You have to eat something," he says sternly. I refuse.

I'm more amenable to his efforts at getting me to walk, because I like to walk, even here. He pushes the wheeled IV stand because it is too heavy for me and holds my hand to help me balance. I feel like the distance between being sick and being healthy is a physical distance, one that I can cover if I just walk far enough.

We make lap after lap of the ward, trying to avoid glancing into any of the rooms, holding our breath at times at some of the smells that even the harsh chemical cleansers can't mask, and edging by the patients lying in beds in the hall while waiting for a room to be free. It doesn't occur to me then how rooms can become free.

I'm in the mood for visitors again, but I don't reinstate

the schedule. Instead, I invite people as I feel like it. Kathie is the first. She's driven all the way from Ithaca, New York, to see me. She's a professor of mycology (the study of fungi) at Cornell University and my oldest friend. I met her in the middle of grade 1 when my family moved to the house where my parents still live today. We did everything together: We scrabbled for fool's gold among the gravel of our school's baseball diamond; we joined a pillow-making class; but most often we played at being orphans escaping from cruel orphanages, making our way in the world alone, and seeking our fortune (a box of crumpled-up balls of aluminum foil).

I was obsessed with orphans. They were my favorite heroes—Anne of Green Gables, Jane Eyre, the girl whose name I forget in *The Wolves of Willoughby Chase*—and my favorite subjects for the plays that I would write or adapt, and that Kathie and I would put on for our admiring parents and bored little brothers in her backyard. Orphans were heroic, tested by tragedy and marked for greatness. I often wondered if I would ever be tested. Would I be brave? Would I leap in front of a bullet, say, to save someone?

When Kathie arrives, she looks fantastic. She's wearing eyeliner, which she doesn't normally wear, and it makes her eyes greener. Long, twisted earrings dangle from her ears, catching the light when she tilts her head to laugh. She laughs a lot. She swings her feet back and forth.

I'm tired. I get short of breath after talking just a little while.

She takes out her phone to show me photos of her new boyfriend. New, new, as in they met the night before and hit it off immediately, one of those dates that begin as coffee, then lunch, then a walk, then dinner, and soon it's twenty-four hours later, and it's love. She's giddy. One of the photos is of their bare feet, leaning in to each other, where the trail pauses and dips down to a waterfall.

I think, now I'll talk, I'll tell her what is going on with me. But how can I do that? I have no way to enter this conversation. It wouldn't be a back and forth. It would be a foreign language, a burst balloon, a cold rainfall. What have I to do with first dates and earrings? I am happy for her, in my mind, I am. It's just my heart that has no room for anything other than me, other than fear. I am that selfish.

I actually banish my brother and my father when, during a visit, they start a lively discussion about Rob Ford, Toronto's then infamous mayor. I'd been in the bathroom for half an hour, returning to face a cold dinner tray. Harish is busy teasing my dad for having voted for Ford. My dad tries to defend himself and then they move on to the next City Hall scandal.

At this point I burst into tears. "I can't do this," I gasp. "I can't talk about this, I can't…" I can't even speak now, I'm sobbing so hard. Harish and my dad scurry out of the room. I'm crying and gulping for breath. My mother tries to be soothing, but her eyes are filling with tears as well.

"It's okay, it'll all be okay," she murmurs. "We're a team. We'll get through this. You need to eat. Please."

For a while, all the gifts lift my spirits. Not only do I receive a constant flow of flowers, gift baskets, books, and cards, but shortly after being admitted I awake from a nap to see thirty beautifully wrapped packages piled on my windowsill, one to open each day of my stay at Sunnybrook. No card is attached. I immediately think of Ann. She was at school with Homer and me and is one of my closest friends. She is so incredibly kind and thoughtful that I assume it must be her. She is silent for a moment on the phone after I spill out my gratitude to her.

"I wish it was me," she says, embarrassed. "I wish I had thought of it. But it wasn't." Now it's my turn to feel bad that I've made her feel bad.

The gifts turn out to be from Peter. He's not going to let me forget this. First I overlooked him as a potential pall-bearer, now this.

In the beginning I open one a day, as directed. The first is a journal, which is so perfect, dusty rose leather with both a ribbon and an elastic to keep your place. It is lined and falls open easily. I use it to record email addresses, phone numbers, Kate's Netflix password that she gave me so I could watch *Downton Abbey*, medication dosages, questions for doctors and their responses, quotes from books I'm reading, even scraps of dialogue I overhear. Even while I'm suffering, part of me is assessing the anecdotal value of everything that's happening to me, thinking this is *great* material.

"Too bad the title *A Heartbreaking Work of Staggering Genius* is already taken," I mourn to Simon.

"Should you really be worrying about titles for your book right now?" he asks.

He's right. I start mentally writing the reviews instead.

Not all the presents are so perfect. One night, nauseous and fatigued from the chemo, but unable to sleep because my throat is so sore that every swallow is a slash of a knife, I open a chess set and a box of peanut brittle.

Finally, one day I'm just so sad I open the last dozen presents all at once. I sit in a sea of torn paper and ribbons, surrounded by silk scarves, organic goat's milk soap, a kit to make little fuzzy felt creatures, a book from the point of view of the servants in *Pride and Prejudice*. It's a distraction and I'm grateful, yet still I weep. I'm not a child at a birthday party. I am a forty-seven-year-old woman chained by an IV line to a hospital bed, wracked with the side effects of induction chemo, and I may not make it.

All these gifts make me think of *The Big C*, a TV series in which Laura Linney plays a mother dealing with a cancer diagnosis. There's an episode where her teenage son, visiting her at the hospital, goes to get her something out of her purse and finds a key with his name and a strange address on it. He goes to the address and it's a storage locker filled with presents, all beautifully wrapped, even a car, all for him: for his sixteenth birthday, his eighteenth birthday, his high school graduation, his college graduation, his wedding. He breaks down, and this is what I think of, will I do this for Jack and Anna? Will I arrange for gifts beyond the grave?

CHAPTER SEVEN

A WEEK AFTER the end of the chemo I start to feel a bit better, right on schedule. I'm done with the fevers it seems, and the blood transfusions have helped. Simon takes me outside for the first time since my admission. I sit in the wheelchair and enjoy the sunshine, but not for long because chemo makes your skin very sensitive so you have to stay out of direct sunlight. It happens to be Mother's Day.

Mother's Day on the Oncology Ward sounds like the title of one of those after-school specials I used to watch as a child on TV in our basement rec room. The ones with improbable calamities and unlikely victories, like the child who sets off firecrackers while skiing, losing both her sight and her legs, but, against all odds, learns both to see and walk again. I don't think they make them anymore. Too cheesy for today's sophisticated youth. Jack and Anna did not even understand that expression when they first heard me using it; unsurprisingly, it happened during a family trip to Florida and involved a giant inflatable shark.

"You mean covered in cheese?" they asked.

They sounded like Simon with his definition of irony: "When your hand gets sore from ironing too much."

So I vow not to shed a tear that day (a big deal because I'm crying every single day at that point) and I manage it because it is just too cliché and over-the-top, movie-of-the-week melo-dramatic to have Mother's Day in a cancer ward, so I refuse to succumb to that, concentrating on concrete steps to get ready.

I take my first shower since being admitted. I have to comb my hair with my fingers though, having thrown out my hairbrush, in a dramatic "I won't be needing this any-more!" moment, only to find that my hair did not fall out as quickly as I had anticipated.

I pick out a fluffy scarf, from the ones friends had given me, that I think best matches the faded blue of my hospital gown. I drape it fetchingly around my neck, trying to hide where the Hickman line sprouts from my chest and attaches me to the IV pump. Then I install myself in the visitors' room next door. I feel that would look nicer than greeting them lying down in a hospital bed.

While my mother and I are waiting for Simon to arrive with Jack and Anna, there are two other visitors in the lounge: a heavy dark-haired man and a skinny woman with inch-thick glasses who does not say a word the whole time but who never stops staring at me.

The man tries to begin a conversation with the pleasant opening of "So, what kind of cancer do you have?"

Without looking at him I say, "I'm sorry but I don't really

feel like talking." So he and the other woman remain silent but still weirdly attentive to our family gathering. I manage to ignore them because I am getting very accomplished at ignoring what I cannot control (which is 99 percent of what seems to be happening to me these days).

At this point, thankfully, Simon and the children arrive. I can't take my eyes off them. I have always held the unbiased belief that they are beautiful, but, in the context of this bleak cancer ward, they seem to be emitting a golden glow of health and happiness and unblemished perfection.

I admire artwork from Anna and a birdhouse Jack made at Scouts. In Jack's card, he lists things I do that he appreciates, including that I "give him neat ideas," which I am surprised by because I had the impression he actively resisted all my suggestions (starting right from grade 2 when he burst into tears because I suggested a slight improvement he could make to his ferret diorama).

When I lose steam, Simon and my mother go to my room to collect some things before taking Jack and Anna home. The woman who had been watching us has, by now, sidled closer and closer, so fascinated does she seem to be with the proceedings. To an outsider, she would look like part of our group. The man has moved closer too, and is now sitting on one side of Jack while I'm on the other.

I hear him ask Jack, "Hey, what's your mother's name?" and Jack tells him.

The man then stands up in front of me and, while my children look on, he says loudly and distinctly, "Manjusha, I am going to pray for you." I couldn't have been more horrified if he had flung out an arm and cursed me.

"Please, not in front of—" I say, gesturing feebly at Jack and Anna, because I'm terrified his next words will be that he is going to pray that I will not die. But he goes on as if I haven't spoken, and repeats, "I am going to pray for you." And then, finally, finally, he exits the room, leaving me shaking and livid, Jack and Anna bemused, and the woman still smiling brightly at us all.

I hated him at that moment and hate him still with an implacable hatred such as I have never felt for anyone else in my life. I think it is because he put in jeopardy all our careful protection of Jack and Anna, and also because he made me feel trapped in a way I have never felt before. I did not have the breath to drown him out and I did not have the strength to leave the room.

I was horrified because I thought his words would make Jack and Anna think I was on my deathbed. Because nobody prays for you unless the situation is dire. If you have the flu or break your leg, people send you a "get well soon!" card and most often a humorous one at that. A *Far Side* fowl with cat-eye glasses and 1950s apron serving her sick son a bowl of chicken soup, saying "Quit complaining, it's nobody we know." But when you have cancer, suddenly you are in everyone's prayers. Even Peter, who is an atheist, told me, "I don't believe in God, but I'm praying for you anyway; let me know how that turns out."

I'm an atheist too, but I'm firmly convinced that if I turn out to be wrong and there is a God, and all the accompanying heaven/hell thing, I am definitely going to heaven. I have no theological basis for this, but I know that it would be ridiculously unfair if I were barred because of what I consider to be a mere technicality, which I equate to the minor procedural irregularities I see in court all the time, and which I either ignore or patch up after the fact in some way. Because, while I do not believe in God, I do believe in justice.

It's silly, I know. Clearly, having a mother who's okay one minute and then hospitalized the next with a diagnosis of cancer has likely worried my children more than anything a random stranger might say. All this eventually does manage to seep into my hysterical brain and I take a deep breath. Jack and Anna seem unfazed, so we chat normally until Simon returns to the room to take them home.

I never stop thinking of my children, not only on Mother's Day, but every single minute of every single day. I try to comfort myself with the cliché that children are our link to immortality, that we continue to live through them. My mother tells me, "You always carry your mother inside of you, no matter what." Or, as I think of it, like I'm Lord Voldemort and Jack and Anna are my Horcruxes. At the very least, they can use this experience to answer the "give an example of how you dealt with adversity" question in their future Harvard applications. So it won't all be for nothing.

One of my favorite doctors has two lines he repeats to me almost every time he sees me and I love them both. The first is about the chemo I am on: "I've never seen this course of treatment fail!" The second is "You'll be dancing at your children's weddings!" The first line fills me with optimism. I have never heard of a doctor being so definite before. This is so great. As almost everyone else in the world will appreciate, not being as naive as I am, there is, sadly, a reason doctors are not usually so definite.

The second line never fails to move me to tears, but they are happy tears. Every word expands to be a promise of a perfect life, the one everyone hopes to have, the one that, before my diagnosis, I took for granted I would have: I will live that long; I will be healthy enough to dance at that advanced age; my children will both get married. He makes me feel like the poor, blind, barren woman in the only fairy tale I ever read where being granted a wish turns out well instead of poorly: She wishes she could lay eyes on her newborn child in its solid gold cradle.

I always used to feel impatient with all those idiots who used up their wishes so stupidly, like the man who wished for a sausage, and finally here is a clever woman who beats the fairy tale odds, and my doctor makes me believe that I can do it too.

CHAPTER EIGHT

"A TEXTBOOK CASE of recovery from chemo!" That's what my doctor tells me I am. "Ordinary and boring," chimes in the hospital pharmacist who often accompanies the doctor on his rounds. I am relieved. In the outside world, individuality is prized; but here in the cancer ward, the last thing you want to be is unique.

They discuss with me the question of whether chemo alone or chemo plus a stem cell transplant would give me the best chance of a permanent recovery. Apparently, it used to be that if you had "good" or "standard" leukemia, you did chemo alone and if you had "bad" leukemia, you did a stem cell transplant. I fall somewhere between "standard" and "bad." But in the last year, Princess Margaret Hospital, the leading cancer hospital in Canada and one of the best in the world, has changed to recommending a stem cell transplant even for standard leukemia. But you have to balance that with the chance that you may not survive the transplant. It is a much riskier treatment than chemo.

At this point, all I know is that getting a stem cell transplant means replacing my immune system with a donor's immune system, since mine was unable to fight my leukemia. There are about 340,000 potential donors on the Canadian stem cell registry, but only about 4 percent are South Asian, and a donor of the same race is more likely to be a genetic match. Many ethnicities are under-represented on the registry. Three-quarters of the potential donors are white. This means my pool of potential donors in Canada is only about 13,600. The Canadian registry is part of a worldwide registry of 24 million people, but still, most of the registries are in Western countries, so the chances of my finding a racial match are low. About 800 people in Canada are waiting for a matching stem cell donor to be found.

My brother is tested and is crushed to find out he's not a match. He's been driving from Waterloo to visit me regularly, bringing take-out food, like sushi and shrimp chips, to tempt me, and writing me weekly letters always including photos of my bright-eyed nieces. He really wanted to be the one to help me.

Even though I don't know yet if I will need a stem cell transplant, and even though I hope I will not need one, I decide I have to get on this now. I feel I must start planning for that extreme contingency. If there's no match for me on the existing registries, I'll have to do some sort of public plea to get more people to sign up. I learn that all it takes to get your genetic information is a cheek swab. And if you're a genetic match for someone, making a donation is similar to giving blood, because stem cells are circulating in your blood. Ten genetic markers are compared to see if someone is a match. Harish was only a 5/10 match and what I need is a 9/10 or 10/10.

It takes weeks to get the results from a cheek swab, and thus it may take months to find a donor, if I find one at all. So even though I don't know if I'll need it, I had better start looking now or it could be too late.

Brampton, a city just outside Toronto where I used to preside, has a large South Asian community. I decide to ask two South Asian lawyers I know, Sonia and Raj, to help me get the word out. I call June to get their contact information. June is my Brampton judicial colleague and friend, but she is more like a fairy godmother. She swooped in when I was first admitted to hospital with flowered pillowcases, organic fruit juices, and homemade meringues. Instead of giving me their emails, she says simply, "Leave it to me."

June calls me back very soon. She has contacted Sonia and Raj, not just to ask people to sign up, but also to organize an actual stem cell drive, where people can give a cheek swab.

"Manjusha!" She always greets me like I'm someone she has been dying to speak to. "Listen, can you call OneMatch? Are you able to? I really think you need to."

OneMatch is the division of Canadian Blood Services that deals with finding stem cell donors. She does not say any more at that point, but gives me the phone number and hints that it will be clear to me what she is up against once I call.

I call and get such a lengthy explanation of the hurdles and the protocols I feel almost a suffocating panic at the thought that OneMatch may not be able to help me. Then, after persisting and asking a few more questions, I learn it is only a matter of my signing some forms to get the process started.

June updates me regularly and I get to witness firsthand what happens when the immovable object of bureaucracy meets the irresistible force of a reformer. June and an army of others have come up with several locations to hold drives, places to reach South Asians—a Hindu temple, a Brampton recreation center, an Indian strip mall. "But OneMatch will only do one drive, that's it," fumes June. "So we have to pick, I think the temple on June the twenty-second would be the best."

Then a few days later, "You won't believe this, but they say there's not enough time to get ready for a drive on the twenty-second, even though we're ready to go; we have the flyers and everything. The earliest they can do is July thirteenth. Something about revising their training materials and the kits won't be ready in time. But Dr. Lala said South Asians 4 Life has at least a hundred kits. I don't know why we can't use theirs, he can do the training." She pauses for breath. "You know, I wanted to check with you first, I don't want to do it without your approval, but I think we need to go higher up in Canadian Blood Services and complain. This is outrageous, it's totally obstructionist, but I'll leave it up to you."

I hesitate. I don't want to seem ungrateful for her passion on my behalf, but I am kind of fixated on my own selfish desire for a stem cell donor and I don't really want to alienate the only organization that's in charge of searching for one for me.

"If it was a three-month delay," I tell June finally, "I'd agree with you, totally...but...since it's only three weeks, maybe, better stay on their good side?" June reluctantly agrees.

"Of course," she says. "That's fine." Though it is not fine at all as evidenced by her next call to me. The problem this time is the realization that July 13 is the day of the World Cup final and there may be many soccer fans among the young South Asian males they're hoping to attract to the drive. But one of the drive organizers says he can make sure there will be a TV at the Hindu Heritage Centre, so people can catch the game; and besides, the drive starts at 11 a.m. and the match isn't until the afternoon, so hopefully it won't even be an issue.

Then it's a problem with tables.

"Manjusha!" June says. "You won't believe this. They say the tables have to be rectangular and the center only has round tables."

"I don't understand," I say, "why does it matter?"

"Oh, something about the volunteer having to be across from the donor while they're explaining the process. I told her we can make sure they sit side by side at the round tables, but it's not good enough."

June calls back to say they managed to find rectangular tables.

"When you've had your transplant, we're going to take this all the way to the top," she fumes. "We're going to rebuild this organization from the ground up. This is unacceptable."

I am relieved. Yes, I agree, absolutely, when I've had my transplant, we'll do all of this. I will help you, I will, when I've had my transplant. If the squeaky wheel gets the grease, but the meek inherit the earth, what providence is there for those of us waiting on endless lists, for stem cells, for organs, for life? At least I don't have to hope for someone to die.

I get to go home right on schedule May 30, exactly thirty days after I was admitted. But there is one last painful procedure before I can leave, a second bone marrow biopsy, to determine how successful the induction chemo was at killing the cancer cells. It's the "You'll dance at your children's wedding" doctor who does it; he's so kind, apologizing for having to go deep into my hip because my bone marrow is "dry" from all the chemo, calling me "love," and asking about Jack and Anna, that he distracts me from the pain. I even manage to ask if he has children. He doesn't, and he adds that he is single, which my brain files away for later.

Then, at last, I'm free to go. I'm clutching my last few belongings in my lap, my pillow and a vaseful of flowers. And Simon starts wheeling me out of the room, when the new patient, who has just moved into the bed next to mine, happens to wake up and I make eye contact with her for the first time. Because I'm in a good mood, I actually stop, say hello, and ask her how she is.

She looks at me dreamily and says, "I'm dying."

And I think to myself, Goddammit, this is exactly why you should never try to start a conversation in a cancer ward. But now I have to pause and think of some response.

I say gently, "You look very peaceful."

She nods and says, "I'm going to God."

I say, "I'm glad."

Then she closes her eyes. I'm not sure if she's asleep, but I think it would be rude to sneak off, so I say quietly, "Well, I'm going home now."

She opens her eyes and says, "I hope you get better before the Rapture."

I say, "Thank you."

And then Simon and I get the hell out of Cancer Ward 2.

CHAPTER NINE

MAKING PANCAKES on the weekend has always been my job. But my first morning at home, Simon makes the pancakes for breakfast. Not only that, but Jack and Anna both pour their maple syrup themselves, even though I'm sitting right there at the table with them. They're in grade 6 and, of course, capable of pouring their own syrup. But the point is, I always did it for them. Anna, in particular, used to make quite the production out of it. She would not even let Simon pour her syrup; it had to be me, because only I could do it exactly right. I've only been gone for a month and everyone has moved on without me.

I'm desperate to be useful, like I used to be. In the hospital I had decided that as soon as I got home, I would buy a gift for the sick child of a friend, whose illness I had heard about while I was at Sunnybrook. Before, I would have felt momentarily terrible but done nothing except enquire periodically about how she was doing. But now, after experiencing the lift of Peter's thirty gifts, I feel I must give her something, but what?

Anna had once received a very soft blanket, which she loved, as a birthday present. I decide on that because I think it would be comforting. Laura is the first friend to visit me at home, so I immediately ask if she'll take me shopping, and she is happy to oblige. When we find the store Anna's blanket was from, I'm crushed to discover they don't have any more in stock. And then I see a rack of stuffed animals at the back of the store, and among them, a very, very soft rabbit with long floppy ears and a sweet expression. This is even better than a blanket. I feel victorious. I carefully compose a card saying that I heard she was going through a hard time, and that I am too, and that I had found comfort in a soft shawl a friend sent me, so I thought she might like this soft rabbit. I arrange for a mutual friend to deliver it.

My next project is to set up one of my doctors with a colleague of mine. It first occurred to me during my last bone marrow biopsy when I learned he was single. I thought it would be weird to propose a blind date from my hospital bed, so the minute I get home, I do it. Because that would not be weird at all.

The fact that I have a spectacularly poor record of matchmaking (June had to suffer through coffee with an academic misanthrope in socks and sandals who called her a Pollyanna), and the fact that he's my doctor, does not deter me in the slightest.

He's reasonably fit, highly intelligent, and very kind. My friend is all of these things, as well as being very pretty—women always have a higher bar to meet. I check with her first and obtain her permission to pass along her email. Then I email him.

Not content merely to suggest they meet, I take it upon myself to suggest restaurant patios they could meet at. Because, of course, a hematologist and a judge cannot be trusted to make a dinner reservation in downtown Toronto, where they both live, without my careful supervision. Maybe I am obsessed with patios because I was confined to a hospital bed just as spring was coming into force. Maybe it's because it's now sunny and warm, and Simon, Jack and Anna, and I are eating all our meals in our backyard, looking out at the ravine in its newly unfurled greenness. It seems really, really important to me that they not eat inside.

In my long email to my doctor, I debate the merits of the rooftop patio at Kensington Kitchen, versus the covered patio at Boulevard Café, both on Harbord Street. I generously suggest all of College Street without confining them to particular restaurants, trusting they cannot go wrong on that strip between Bathurst and Christie.

I do manage to refrain from suggesting that I can perform their wedding ceremony.

I'm feeling so good after I get home that I start to fantasize, and then, dangerously, really believe, that all this has been a mistake—that when Simon and I go on June 5 to get the results from the bone marrow biopsy, my doctor will tell me that not only do I not have leukemia anymore, but that I never had it in the first place. It sounds foolish, but truthfully, isn't that what we all really long for? Not simply to be cured, but not to have been sick in the first place? So why do we only voice a wish for what is possible? Why don't we go ahead and wish for what we really want?

On June 3, Simon and I attend a Princess Margaret Hospital informational session about stem cell transplants. My doctor managed to arrange it for us even though the transplant team normally meets with you only when you have a donor. Homer gave me questions ahead of time to ask about the efficacy of stem cell transplants, which I carefully read out to them from my journal:

Do you have a large randomized study of people like me on the long-term outcomes of chemo alone versus chemo plus stem cell transplant?

If not, do you have a reasonable belief that one is better than the other?

How do you weigh a small risk of a catastrophic outcome?

The simple answer to the first and biggest question is, no, they do not have any clear-cut studies. One of the transplant team residents tells me that if I'm in the high-risk genetic subgroup, it is clear-cut that a transplant is better than chemo alone. If I am in the favorable genetic subgroup, chemo alone is better. But I'm not in either of these groups. I'm somewhere in between, though leaning toward higher risk. But they see me as a strong candidate for the procedure, and they could do it as early as mid-July if I can find a donor. It seems to come down to simply this: If you have a donor, you do a transplant; if you don't have a donor, you do chemo alone.

A successful stem cell transfer would increase my chances

of surviving from 50 percent (which is the rate with chemo alone) to 65 percent. In medical terms this is a huge gain. The bad news is that it involves another six-week stay in hospital with another round of chemo (more aggressive even than the one I just had), followed by radiation to make sure my own immune system is absolutely killed off. Then they transplant the new immune system.

The six weeks in hospital is followed by an eighteen-month recovery period and during the whole time they are watching carefully that this new immune system does not attack and kill me (it is meant to attack only any residual leukemia cells, but it might also perceive my own organs as invaders). The chances of the transfer killing me are 10 to 15 percent, yet doing it only increases my chances of survival by 15 percent. I run all this by Homer and he thinks I must have misheard, because if those were really the odds then it would not make sense to risk the transplant—yet the hospital is recommending it. Maybe I did misunderstand. Probability and statistics is the only course I ever got a C in, and it's way harder to process the risk when it concerns your own life and death.

I never contemplated that the road to recovery would be more than two years long before I returned to work. I had not pictured that Jack and Anna would go from almost twelve to almost fourteen before I returned to them as I was before. I had not (in my childish optimism) realized that when they had been offering me a cure all this time, they had not meant they were handing me my life back (which is what I had thought) but rather they were handing me a lottery ticket.

I decide to put the idea of a stem cell transplant completely

out of my mind. Since it is out of my control I will not think
of it. Instead, I'm going to concentrate on the fact that so far
I'm doing well with the chemo alone. I've got the cruise we
booked for my parents' fiftieth wedding anniversary in the
second week of December to look forward to, and I spend the
day before my appointment on the phone with a travel agent
sorting through various options for other trips. I find it overwhelming to search for things on the Internet. I always prefer
speaking to a live person, so I start with the tour company I
used for my trip to Africa. I want Africa again, but the agent
tells me October and July are the best times to see the migra-
tions across the Serengeti and those times don't work for me,
so instead I ask about Costa Rica.

She wants to know how I heard about their tours. My
favorite question! I launch into the story of how Simon and I
met on one of their tours in Africa and how now, fifteen years
later, we want to go again, but this time with our eleven-year-
old twins. She loves the story. I offer to do an infomercial for
them. She laughs and I laugh too, to show I was totally kidding. I wasn't.

Simon and I go to see Anna in her opera company's pro-
duction of *East of the Sun, West of the Moon* at Harbourfront.
I get to revel in all the witches, enchanted bears, and danc-
ing trolls that have been missing in my life this last month.
We eat a dim sum lunch at a restaurant overlooking the lake.
Then Simon pushes me in a wheelchair along the boardwalk
even though the wind off the water is cold. I can walk, but
I'm weak after a month in hospital.

I can picture my own magical moment so clearly. The
doctor will admit his mistake in his usual charming, low-key

manner. We will all have a good chuckle about it. And because I like and respect him (hey, anyone can make a mistake) and because I will be so relieved, I will not even think of suing him or by extension the hospital. I think this is pretty noble of me.

Then the bunny returns. Not literally, but my friends send me a grateful email thanking me for thinking of their child, especially while immersed in my own struggle, but, and this is a big but, regretfully telling me she would not want to have people treat her differently, to have people know something is wrong.

My attempt at matchmaking fails as well. Surprisingly, to me that is, though not to anyone else, the doctor never responds to my email suggesting that patio date.

Instead of seeing these small failures as a sign of larger ones to come, I arrive with Simon for my appointment, wearing something pretty for the first time in a month—a short striped skirt and peach-colored sweater—and clutching a list of questions, the first of which is whether I can go snorkeling in Costa Rica this winter.

The consultant arrives, with a nurse in tow, pulls up a little stool to sit on, and tells us the biopsy results.

The induction chemo has not been successful.

I still have leukemia.

He explains that he had not expected to get the percentage of leukemia cells in my blood completely down to zero, but that a successful induction means that the proportion of cancer cells is down to less than 5 percent, and the biopsy showed an amount slightly over that, somewhere between 5 and 10 percent. I just missed the cutoff.

Homer explains to me later that the cutoff is arbitrary in that a few percentage points past it may have been okay, but they have to have a cutoff. Still, this means instead of moving on to the consolidation chemo sessions, I have to do another month in hospital for another round of induction chemo, but now at five times the strength of the first round, and with three types of chemo instead of two. The third type is to weaken the enzyme in my genetic mutation that is preventing the chemo from entering the cancer cells.

The words "drug transport through cellular membrane" pop into my mind. I've copyedited that line. My mother was doing her PhD in biochemistry at the University of Toronto when I was in high school. I used to proofread her papers for her. Her research was about the ability of certain drugs to pass through cell membranes. I didn't understand then what I was reading. My job was to insert all the missing articles of speech, the *the*s and *a*s that the Marathi language does not use and that my mother always left out. My only questions were along the lines of "Is it *the* membrane or *any* membrane?" I didn't care which, I just needed to know. Now I care.

This second induction round will involve FLAG-something chemotherapy. I don't know what the acronym stands for, but I picture a battle flag being replaced with a white one of surrender. My particular leukemia is proving chemo-resistant, which means future relapse is more likely than not. Instead of a 50 percent chance of being cured with chemo, I am down to a 40 percent chance. And that means a stem cell transplant is most probably the way to go.

This particular FLAG regime is fairly new; my doctor tells me that so far it has been given only five times at Sunnybrook, and ninety-five times at Princess Margaret. I am healthy otherwise, so I'm considered a good candidate for it. We listen to a description of how very toxic it will be. There will be worse side effects than before, a chance of ending up in the Intensive Care Unit, a chance of death even. I will be very, very sick.

Simon has his head down; much later he tells me he thought he was going to pass out, he was so shocked. We felt caught off guard. It hadn't even occurred to us that this was a possibility, that the first round of chemo could fail. We didn't even twig to the fact that the doctor had a nurse with him when he spoke to us, something he doesn't normally do, to help us cope with the news.

Because I don't want to be caught so off guard again, I ask what the next treatment would be if the second induction also fails.

The answer is, nothing.

And I think, no, no, no. Yet again, the doctors are not following the right script. I know people who've gone through this, I've seen the movies, I've read *The Fault in Our Stars*. You can torture people with treatment options for years, *years!* Surgery, radiation, clinical trials, experimental drugs. Do it to me! Surely I can't reach the end of the line thirty days after being diagnosed with leukemia.

The doctor is calm. He says he believes this chemo will work. But if it doesn't work, it means I'm not in remission. If I'm not in remission, I'm not a candidate for stem cell transplant. Even if I'm lucky enough to find a donor, I can't do a transplant if I still have leukemia in me. So what I thought was such a terrifying option now feels like something I can only dream of being lucky enough to try.

When the doctor leaves to see his next patient, the nurse stays with us. He is kind, gentle, soft-spoken. He wants to know if there's anything he can do, if there is anything we need. Simon points out to me later that he is my soft rabbit. Now I understand. Sometimes a soft rabbit is not just a soft rabbit, but a sign, a scarlet letter, a portent of doom.

And so we leave. I feel ugly and sad and defeated. All along I was just worried about the cancer coming back at some point in the near or distant future. It did not occur to me for one moment that they would not be able to get rid of it in the first place. It did not enter my mind because I felt so good! It's like that relationship quip, "How can I miss you, if you won't go away?" That's how I feel. How can I even get to the point of worrying about the cancer returning if it won't leave in the first place? How could I be so worried and then find out that I wasn't even worried enough? I thought I was scared before. That was nothing.

Now

I

Am

Scared.

Is this a lesson for me, to appreciate the days I have, to stop and smell the roses? But I don't need a lesson. I already left no rose unsmelled. Seeing a cardinal *always* made me happy no matter how frequently I saw one in a single day. A pair lives in our backyard, and another pair lives a few houses away, so they're not exactly a rare spotting.

Instantly I change my mind about my silly image of being first in line, about needing to take my turn. I decide I did not need this; I did not deserve this; no one deserves this. But to my cry of "Why?" the universe just shrugs its shoulders and says "Why not?" Fair enough. Why not me, after all? Yes, I didn't deserve it, but I didn't deserve all the good I got either. It works both ways.

I had thought I controlled everything that happened, to me, to my family, to the litigants who appeared in front of me. My own mother-in-law feels she has to apologize when she uses too many exclamation marks in emails to me because she knows I will disapprove. I was upset when it rained for most of the week we were in Mexico the January before my diagnosis because I was miffed to discover that there was actually something—weather!—that was beyond my control. Now I'm learning what a fantasy I was living; there is nothing within my control.

Simon says simply, "They will get the leukemia with this round." He reminds me that they are still saying this is the plan to cure me.

Homer says to focus on two things only:

1. Your job is to get better, period.

2. Do not admit the possibility of failure, as you have never failed at anything you ever tried before.

On Saturday, Simon, Simon's mom, Jack, and I drive up north to collect Anna from her Music by the Lake camp and we get to hear her symphony orchestra perform. The camp is for middle school students and they have been practicing four hours every day for a whole week and then listening to the professional faculty play concerts every night. They start with Vivaldi's *Spring* and from the first beautiful note, perfectly in tune, unlike any other school concert we have ever been to, I am blown away by all of it: the swell of the oh-so-familiar music; the blue sky; Anna's earnest bow strokes; the benches crowded with family members.

We run into several of our camping friends after the concert. Their teenage daughters, Liora and Ella, hang back while we chat, but as we say goodbye they both hug me, not something they would normally do, and it brings tears to my eyes because it is tender, it is close, and it says what they cannot: I hope you'll be okay.

I'm tired from the morning and our car is quite a distance away from where we're eating our hot dog lunch. Simon asks one of the camp directors if he can bring our car up to the picnic tables and the director offers instead to drive me to the parking lot. In the brief drive, he speaks about his wife, who also has trouble walking very far, and his voice catches as he describes how sick she is. In a strange way it comforts me by reminding me, again, that I am not alone.

There's a Hindu fable about a man who goes to the gods for help for his seriously ill son; he is begging for a cure. The gods say, Sure we'll help, provided, that is, you bring us a handful of salt from a house in your village that has never known sorrow.

CHAPTER TEN

BARELY A WEEK after my escape, I find myself installed right back in Cancer Ward 2, or Hotel California, as I start to call it. You can be discharged anytime you like, but you can never leave. While I'm worried about what's to come, uppermost in my mind is that it would be easier to face the extra-toxic chemo than the doctor I tried to set up with my friend. I confide my feeling of awkwardness to a couple of the female members of my medical team, a resident and one of the nurses, and that immediately makes me feel better.

"Oh my god," they chorus. "We've been trying to set him up for years, he's so stubborn and picky. Your friend sounds great. We'll get right to work on him, don't worry." Word of my plotting spreads (as these things do) and another member of my team drops by my bedside to chat and reveals that he has recently been through a breakup and would love to meet someone.

"I'm totally on it," I tell him. And I do have just the person for him to meet, but I tell him I have to wait until Monday to contact her because I only have her work number not her home number (she's a lawyer who used to appear regularly in front of me—again not weird at all—and I never do end up contacting her). So now some of my medical team drops by to gossip about relationships, which I love, and the subject of my genetic mutations does not even come up.

I try to focus on the fact that, despite all the attendant risks, my team seems confident that this regime will put me in remission.

My friend Vineet told me I should tell the universe what I want. So this is my positive message to the universe:

At the end of this month, June 2014, I will achieve remission.

At the end of the next month, July 2014, I will find an exact-match stem cell donor and I will have a successful transplant.

Eighteen months after that, January 2016, I will be back in court.

In July 2016, Simon, Jack, Anna, and I will be standing on the Serengeti plain watching the migration of millions of wildebeests and zebras.

And in 2047, when I am eighty and looking back on my life, I will call this two-year struggle a "worthwhile lesson" rather than a "hellish ordeal."

I was so caught by surprise this week to be told that this second induction chemo is the last treatment option they have for me that I resolve to prepare myself better for the future. So I enquire about other options. In Ottawa, they will do a stem cell transplant even if you are not in remission, so long as you have a donor. In Vancouver, they will do a transplant using umbilical cord blood. I don't know if I can use the cord blood we banked after Jack and Anna's birth. In Hamilton, they will do a transplant with a half match (a 5/10, which is what my brother was) as long as you are in remission.

My friend Lois from law school who now works at Johns Hopkins University in Philadelphia contacts me with information about some clinical trials in the United States. They are also experimenting with things like stem cell transplants with a half match. It seems much scarier though to think of going to the States. Because it is a trial, the drugs are covered by the company administering them, but you have to pay your own hospital and other medical expenses and there are the travel costs and the accommodation costs of whoever is accompanying you. It would bankrupt you, I think. Plus, I was told at my information session at Princess Margaret Hospital that a half match (or mismatch, as they more forebodingly call it) increases your risk of dying from the transplant itself from 15 percent to 30 percent. That seems way too high.

When I call the ward the day before my admission this time around to make sure there is a bed available, the nurse asks me if I want a private room. "Absolutely!" I say. I'm delighted because I didn't think that was even a possibility. But it's clearly some kind of mix-up because when Simon and I arrive on the morning of my admission, not only is there no private room, they ask if I would mind sharing a room with two men, because the alternative would be a bed in the corridor. I pitied those corridor patients during my first month, their belongings in piles around them, subject to the lights and the noise all through the night, with patients edging by with walkers or wheelchairs, and nurses and doctors and residents rushing past. So I say "Fine" and regret it immediately.

The first man is much older than I am and moans and complains constantly, while the other man who is around my age burps (and worse). The noises I hear from the bathroom make me avoid it entirely, even though it means dragging my IV stand down the hall to the toilet in the shower station.

"You never visit," the first man accuses his wife, almost every time she visits.

"I've been here every day."

"You only stayed a few minutes."

"I was here for four hours, you were asleep the whole time."

By this time they are glaring at each other. And yet there she is the next day and they go through it all again. I decide I wouldn't bother if I were her.

The second man is on the phone fighting with his insurance company all day. Whenever we make eye contact, we just look at each other, neither one of us smiles. Two nurses with mops once rush in to clean our bathroom and tell me, "Don't use the bathroom for a few hours!"

"Don't worry," I answer, "I've never used it and I never

plan to!" After four days I am moved to a two-person room with a quiet woman. I don't have a window, but that is the least of my concerns this time around.

"CBC Radio wants to do a documentary about you!" Kate is excited. I'm not so sure. Do I have the energy in the middle of chemo to speak to a reporter, I wonder. Shouldn't I be concentrating on surviving my treatment? But I don't want to seem ungrateful. This is the result of Kate's unflagging efforts to spread the word about my search for a stem cell donor. She has been contacting every person who has ever known me. The CBC reporter, Alisa, was immediately interested because she knew me from a story she'd done about an international adoption I presided over. I decide I should say yes and before I know it Alisa is at Sunnybrook to record the first of several interviews.

"I have a few questions," she tells me smilingly when we meet, "but really I just want you to talk about how you're doing—tell me stories." And so I talk. I talk about being scared, I talk about Jack and Anna. She interjects only occasionally. "What music do you listen to?" she asks when I tell her about how I rely on a borrowed iPod to block out all the noise in the ward. I mention Jim Cuddy, because I try to imagine, along with him, that I have a skyscraper soul, "with mud in my veins and steel in my bones." She loves that and begs me to sing those lines for her into her microphone, but I refuse. There is only so much I am prepared to do to get a stem cell donor.

She says I gave her gold. "I could do a five-hour Manjusha show if they would give me the time," she gushes. That makes Simon laugh when I tell him, because his life is nonstop listening to the Manjusha show.

A member of my medical team is there at the beginning of the interview, though he tells Alisa he doesn't want to be taped. He tells her that when he first saw my name written next to this extra-strong chemo regime, he wept. And he tears up even as he is speaking about it. At first I am surprised and touched, but after contemplating it further, I decide my doctor's no-nonsense approach, that this is just the next thing we recommend to cure you, even with the statistical risk in play, is better than scaring me with tears. Since statistics are cold, and since I don't really understand them, I don't think about them. But seeing a professional cry because they feel sorry for you would alarm anyone. His tears scare me more than the actuarial risk of death I face. I can't help thinking it must be dire if members of my medical team are weeping for me; the next thing you know they'll be praying for me, and then for sure I'll know the end is nigh.

Alisa and I start off in the visitors' room as there is no one else in there, when a nursing manager and some hospital communications people come bustling in and admonish me for not clearing the interview with them first, which never occurred to me. They're accommodating enough in the end though, even finding us a small closet in which to have the interview. It cannot be in my room in order to protect my roommate's privacy, though Alisa really wants ambient hospital noise (the IV alarms would have come in useful for once). One of them even gets quite chatty, mentioning helpfully that her niece, age twelve, died waiting for a stem cell donor that was never found.

Meanwhile, Kate keeps my spirits up with constant updates about all the stem cell drives that are happening, in addition to the big one planned in Mississauga on July 13. My uncle in Scotch Plains, New Jersey; my friend Kathie in Ithaca, New York; my aunt in Pune, India, are also organizing drives. Even the Asian American Donor Program, an incredible organization, is planning a drive for me in Milpitas, California.

My plea for a stem cell donor has been published in a newsletter for all the Marathi organizations in North America (someone from Maharashtra, India, would be my likeliest match). This newsletter is also sent to all Marathi households (some 1,200) in Toronto. There have been stories about my search in several South Asian newspapers, magazines, TV and radio shows, and in the *Toronto Star*.

Kate has been urging people to go to my Facebook page, which she created, to share it and like it and add comments to it, because the more activity on the page, the more people will see it, and the more likely they will be to go to onematch.ca or to an event to register. Even people who are not in the target ethnicity or age range may know someone who is. When Kate finds out that blood donations in Canada are at a five-year low, she urges people to give blood as well. And Alisa's documentary, *Manjusha's Match*, ends up airing nationally multiple times.

I'm going to need an awful lot of people to sign up. Only one in three hundred people on the registry will end up being a match for someone, and not a match for me particularly, but a match for someone, somewhere, in the world.

And then, on June 19, 2014, Senator Asha Seth makes the following statement in the Senate in Ottawa, which I don't hear about until well after the fact:

Hon. Asha Seth: Honorable senators, it is a tragedy when our citizens suffer through no fault of their own. This is the case of Madam Justice Manjusha Pawagi, a wife and mother of twins who is currently in the fight of her life against a rare type of leukemia.

You may have heard of this highly accomplished 47-year-old who is also an award-winning children's book author, a Stanford-educated journalist and, since 2009, a Brampton-based family judge. If she makes it through her second month-long round of chemo, she has only a 50 percent chance of survival.

However, her chances could be significantly increased through a simple procedure known as a stem cell transfusion.

Unfortunately, in the South Asian community, and in many minority groups, there are very low rates of blood and stem cell donations, making the chances of finding genetic matches more than one in a million due to lack of diversity in the blood and stem cell supply. This lack of participation is reflected in the Canadian Blood Services' reports, which show that more than 70 percent of their donors are Caucasian.

Establishing stem cell registries that reflect the diversity of the Canadian population is crucial because stem cells have an incredible ability to develop into many other types of beneficial cells, and in treating over seventy diseases worldwide.

It is imperative that we encourage our entire population, and especially minority groups, to register today with a blood and stem cell registry such as Canada's onematch.ca.

Justice Pawagi is just one of the thousands of people in our country and around the world who wait with a very heavy heart for a donor, a savior, a hope to regain their health.

It is not too late for Justice Pawagi and I hope to bring a positive change in this case, but I need your support in spreading this urgent message for others.

Apparently some government official had read the newspaper article about me and it got passed up the government chain until it reached the Senate itself. Simon thinks I shouldn't mention this Senate speech.

"People won't be able to relate," he says and I can totally see his point. The average person in my situation does not get a mention in the Canadian parliament's upper chamber. But I think the whole question of privilege and power is an important one and I should address it head on, not hide it. Why am I getting all this attention?

Is it "connections"? The word has such negative connotations as it conjures up private schools and country clubs. But my connections are exactly what the word means, people I'm connected to, in other words, my friends. Homer, now a surgeon at Sunnybrook, who is helping me navigate and understand the medical jargon and treatment plans, I met in grade 7 when he was a chess-club-joining, violin-playing eleven-year-old. Scott, now at the *Toronto Star*, was the partying, news editor charmer of the student paper where as an undergrad I was a features editor. I met Kathie, who organized a drive for me at Cornell University where she is a professor, when we were six years old.

Is it because I'm a judge? Kate told me she was uncomfortable putting that fact in any of the outreach messages or posters. However, one of the South Asian lawyers helping to organize the drive told her that fact would get more people out because it was something people in the community were proud of—that one of them had attained a position of prominence—and would galvanize them. I think I'm the first South Asian family court judge in Ontario. And yet the "Principles of Judicial Conduct" I had hanging outside my office door state that it is inappropriate for judges to engage in fundraising activities because it would be an improper use of their considerable influence, and here I am asking not for money, but for blood!

Is it because I'm the mother of two young children? To me this is my biggest hook because it is what I would be most moved by. So I guess you could say I "used" my children. The photo I give for all the drives (and everyone wants a photo) is one of me with my arms around Jack and Anna, who are both leaning into me and smiling winningly at the camera, with a backdrop of flowers in the Montreal Botanical Garden. I want to tug at heartstrings, I want people to think, Oh those beautiful children, how could they be left motherless?

I used to love medical dramas on TV, like *ER* and later *House*. But I cared only about patients who had loved ones gathered at their bedsides. To me the tragedy was not death itself, because once you were dead there was no more suffering, there was nothing. The tragedy was in the heartache you left behind, because that would go on and on.

Still I'm troubled. I fear that all I'm doing is rationalizing my privilege. My request is self-interested, period. I'm reaching out only because I desperately need a match. Would I be asking otherwise? No, because I had never even heard of stem cell transplants or the stem cell registry until I got sick. But still, it's not like people are depositing their cheek swabs directly in my mailbox, I tell myself. All I'm asking is for more people to sign up on the registry. Not only is it a public Canadian registry, but it's connected to a global registry. The people who sign up because of my plea could end up helping me or someone else anywhere in the world. And because of that I decide I don't feel guilty about the media attention and all the drives my friends are organizing. I'm helping more people than just myself. And I find that comforting. If I don't make it, I will at least have increased the chances of someone else surviving.

At any given time almost a thousand people in Canada, and thousands more around the world, are desperate to find a stem cell match. I promise myself that if I make it, I will continue to campaign for people to get swabbed and on the registry. I won't stop because I'm safe. Some countries in Europe have huge registries because of their opt-out system. They seek to swab everyone, and you actually have to say no, in order to stay off the registry. Germany's population is only a little more than double Canada's, and yet it has five and a half million people on its registry, *eighteen times* the number we have on ours. We should have that in Canada, instead of our current system of relying on individual pleas for donors. We should find a way to reach every possible donor. It could be something as simple as asking every student to give a cheek swab as they leave high school. Maybe that could be my calling. One day. When I am better.

During my interview with Alisa, she asks me what in my life prepared me to face this ordeal. And my answer, at first, is nothing. Absolutely nothing. I have had a soft, easy life with no hardships whatsoever. While I have worked hard, now that I can no longer work at all, I see the ability to work hard as a gift, rather than a hardship. I'm desperate to get back to the job I loved so much. Friends tell me I'll get through this because I'm strong. This is kind, but untrue. I'm probably the weakest person I know. I think maybe it's gratitude that has prepared me. I have never taken for granted what I have, but have always been very grateful for it.

It makes me think happiness is mostly a choice you make, not a state you're in. I remember growing up and my parents referring to us as being "upper middle class." I see now that of course we were not upper middle class, just ordinary middle class. But because my parents felt rich, they made me feel rich. In the children's novel *Kira, Kira* the family falls apart when the older sister dies of cancer, the father has a meltdown at work and loses his job, and it all seems to go from bad to worse. But then they hit a turning point when he realizes that they have a choice: They can choose to be a happy family.

CHAPTER ELEVEN

MY INTEREST in matchmaking ends gradually as the chemo starts to accumulate in my blood and I sink into myself. I was enjoying dissecting the recent breakup of one of my medical team members: What went wrong? Is there a chance they can get back together based on what she recently texted him? I'm flattered and pleased with my identity as relationship guru, as opposed to sad little cancer patient. But when the full effect of the chemo hits me, I start to feel uneasy and dreamlike. I feel like I belong more elsewhere than where I actually am. Like I'm a hummingbird, the only creature, according to North American legend, granted the ability to go back and forth between this world and the next. Like I can hover over both and be part of neither.

The specially certified chemo nurses come in briskly each day, stripping off their regular blue gloves and putting on special yellow chemo gloves before they attach the bags to my

IV pump. They then throw out the yellow gloves in a special trash can before exiting my room. Meanwhile, the drugs they can't touch, even through a plastic bag and with special gloves, are traveling directly into my veins for seven hours each day. This treatment could kill me before the cancer gets a chance to.

I'm so sad and so nauseous and so scared that I don't have the mental energy to care about anyone else. I can barely muster up the energy to call Jack and Anna each night to hear about their day; I no longer have the strength to be embarrassed about my matchmaking attempts; I can no longer listen to my team member babble on about his failed relationship and so I selfishly pretend to be asleep every time he comes into my room.

As a long-stay patient I have learned that a hospital is not a bricks and mortar building but an alternative world, a netherworld of pain and sickness and suffering. I was once bumped from getting a CT scan because an urgent motorcycle accident victim took priority. I tried not to look, but I couldn't help but see the blood, hear his agony, and sense the terror of his wife sitting beside me for hours in the only chair outside the procedure room.

The gore makes it sound medieval, but it is actually a futuristic world of miraculous machines and incredible feats and troops and troops of top-notch professionals. Only these workers can travel between this netherworld and the real world. They are the real hummingbirds. At times it is the real world that seems unreal to me. I cannot picture that there are people out there, working, playing soccer, sending back dishes at restaurants. To comfort me, a friend says that afterwards, this will all be a blur. But I hope I don't forget, because I think I'll be a more thoughtful person if I can remember, always, that this netherworld exists.

Comedy is supposed to be tragedy plus time, but my tragedy and comedy are racing to keep up with each other, and the relief of writing my posts on CaringBridge is such that I soon catch up and have no time left in which to transform my pain.

JUN 13, 2014 7:32 AM:

Forget everything I ever wrote that made me seem brave or accepting or sweetly resigned. It's all crap, my sad attempt to continue to please, to win praise, etc. I can put up a hopeful—or in the sad alternative— a resigned front for most of the daylight hours. But then in that hour before bedtime, especially if Jack and Anna have just visited, like they did last night, and chattered all about their upcoming grade 6 graduation ceremonies, and how I'm the best mummy in the world (Anna), and how they don't want to leave yet, and can't they go back and see my room one more time (Jack), I am crushed.

I am crushed by a wave of guilt so huge that I can barely breathe. I lie there and weep and think it is incredibly tragic and ironic or whatever, that I, who have only ever wanted my children to be happy, and I who have done everything I could to make them so, am going to be solely responsible for heaping on them a sadness such as no young child should have to experience, a grief that will stay with them their entire lives. I will not be there for them for all the things they will need me for in the years and years to come. And I know technically this is not my fault— it is random bad luck—but I am the instrument, I am the one who will have left them and it feels like it is all my fault.

Everything Simon and I did was for them. And we tried so hard especially to make them realize how beautiful this world is. We've taken them to England and Mexico half a dozen times. We've explored London, Paris, and New York City with their beloved cousins Hannah, Nick, and Juliet and Uncle George and Aunt Michele. Some of our magical moments have been seeing animals in the wild, something so unexpected and unplanned it sweeps you away. We saw a blue whale in the St. Lawrence, mountain caribou in the Gaspé peninsula, mother and baby moose in Algonquin. Jack would drag me out of bed at 6 a.m. at the cottage to go bird watching, and though I grumbled, I braved the mosquitoes and was as thrilled as he was when we saw a pileated woodpecker (think Woody Woodpecker with a great big red crest). This summer we had a big trip booked to England, Wales, and Amsterdam (the latter was Simon's great idea). We had listened to Anne Frank's diary on CD in the car and were all so moved by it. We thought it would be really something to show them the secret annex where she hid for two whole years. We wanted to inspire them and move them—and above all bring them joy. We've spent every Easter weekend since they were two years old with Kathie in Ithaca, hunting Easter eggs, looking for fossils, and hiking. We've had wonderful Winterludes in Ottawa with Kate and her incredibly precious family, especially this last time where the highlight was all eight of us holding hands and zipping down the family ice slide, bumping into each other and shrieking with laughter.

Any of you who have seen my chambers know it is a Jack and Anna gallery of their artwork and photos (mummy and me in Mexico, in the Dominican, cuddling on the sofa). I've managed to include things they've written in speeches I've given. Apologies to those who have already heard this…when Anna was six she wrote me a story for Mother's Day that told how I got Jack and Anna. Apparently I won them in a loveliness contest. I and a few other women were walking down the street when we saw two babies on the sidewalk, and we had to decide who would get to keep them. So we had a contest. The categories were who's the prettiest, who's the nicest and I won all the categories, and so got to keep the babies. I thought what the story really showed was more what she felt about herself than what she felt about me. She felt so secure and loved that there was no doubt in her mind that she and her brother were so precious that the ultimate prize would be the privilege of looking after them forever.

And now it may be that I am going to lose that privilege and it is NOT fair and it is NOT right because I did not take it for granted for one single second. I did try so hard to deserve this very great privilege. And even though I am not going to say this to them, I still want them to know somehow that I am so very, very, very, very sorry to be the reason for making them so sad.

I am so sorry.

Simon is completely appalled when he reads this post. The first words out of his mouth when he sees me the next day are "Have you lost your mind? What the hell were you thinking?"

I remind him that I had told him I was starting to get too tired to post, and he was the one who urged me to put up at least something every day so I had a record of my experience.

He responds, a little testily, I think, that he meant I should be posting a record of how I was handling chemo, not a premature goodbye to Jack and Anna.

So we agree to disagree; or, more accurately, I agree to let him vet my posts until I can be trusted to post responsibly and not scare away all my CaringBridge supporters.

"The bathroom is for patients only!" I remind my roommate when I notice that her adult son has used our bathroom. There's a giant, brightly colored sign on the door saying that. Bathrooms for visitors are by the elevators. I've been keeping a beady eye on her side of the room, where the bathroom is, because she has a lot of visitors, including a toddler grandchild, and I'm suspicious that they're going to use the bathroom. And so when one of them does, I interject immediately.

"I'm immunosuppressed!" I remind her. "I can get sick so easily. Visitors have to use the bathroom down the hall."

"My son, he's Greek," she apologizes. "He can't read English so well." Which is ridiculous. Since her English is fine and she has only a slight Greek accent, I'm pretty sure her grown children are fluent in English.

We get along well otherwise. When I see that she's struggling to eat, despite all the nurses do to urge her, I try to encourage her by telling her what I do.

"I try to eat something every hour," I tell her, "even if it's only a little bit." I had saved my bread and butter and small packet of strawberry jam from lunch and I was eating it as an afternoon snack, when I overhear her tell the nurse that I told her to take at least one bite every day.

"Not every day," I correct from my side of the curtain, "every *hour!*"

Simon and I go to one of the hospital cafés for lunch the next day and I optimistically order two hot dogs (I end up not even finishing one). I normally don't eat hot dogs, but I order them because it reminds me of Music by the Lake and the hot dogs that were served there by the water's edge, in the sunshine. It's sunny today as well, and Simon takes me for a ride outside in my wheelchair.

Simon blames the hot dog. But I think it started with

the popcorn. Even my darkest hours begin and end with snacks. I was eating a small bag of popcorn as my bedtime snack that night (because I was in hospital I thought I should have something healthier than Cheetos), rereading *Wave*, a memoir by a woman who lost her whole family—two young sons, husband, both parents—to a tsunami in Sri Lanka. When Simon saw me pack it in my hospital bag he wanted to know, what, there were no memoirs about the Holocaust or the Rwandan genocide available at the library that day? But I've always found it inspiring to read about people worse off than me. During relationship breakups my go-to was always Amy Tan's *The Kitchen God's Wife*. There's nothing like that to put the tragedy of "He's not that into you" in perspective. He may not return my calls, I would think, but at least he didn't lure me into thinking I was going to be an honored wife rather than an enslaved concubine. I have often thought I would love the job of prescribing books to people for what ails them, like in the book *Novel Cure*. Or like Lucy's stall in *Peanuts*, but for literature rather than psychiatry. I can picture my sign: The Book Doctor is IN.

I take a second bag of popcorn out of my closet shelf and settle back down with my book. I feel a stabbing pain in my stomach. I shift uncomfortably, but continue to nibble on my popcorn. It comes again, and this time the pain doesn't stop. I buzz for a nurse. When she comes, it's someone I've never seen before. I ask for more pain medication. She leaves but then returns empty-handed. "You had your last dose one hour ago, you can't have your next dose for another hour."

The pain is searing.

"I can't wait that long," I whimper.

She looks at me unsympathetically. "You're eating pop-corn," she points out in an accusing tone. Through my haze of pain I'm not sure what the accusation is, exactly. That if you're well enough to snack you must not be that sick? She goes away.

I buzz again immediately. When she returns I beg her to ask the doctor to give me my next dose of pain medication early.

She presses her lips together. "The doctor is not here."

"Call him!" I wail. She reluctantly agrees and leaves.

I buzz again the second she's gone. I no longer know what I'm doing. I have never been in such agony. I'm clutching my stomach and I'm moaning with pain. And then I'm scream-ing. But even as I scream, I'm feeling guilty. You're disturbing everyone on the ward, I tell myself. There are a lot of sick people here, they don't need to hear this. But I can't help it. I keep screaming and screaming. And then.

Nothing.

CHAPTER TWELVE

MOST PEOPLE in my situation wouldn't think of calling a press conference, but I'm pretty proud of myself for thinking of it. It's risky, I know, but I have to reveal everything I have discovered about Sunnybrook, even though I'm still trapped here in its Intensive Care Unit. Luckily, there's a thick glass window at the foot of my hospital bed separating me from the crowds that have gathered in the hallway outside my room. They seem hostile, jostling against each other as the space gets more and more packed. Many of them are carrying weapons. I am relieved to see that when Simon and the kids finally arrive, Jack and Anna are being shielded by my friend Sharon's sons, Cole with his BB gun and Noah with his homemade knife.

Doctors are pretending to be nurses, nurses are pretending to be doctors. Not to mention that the ICU itself has been outsourced to the middle of the Canadian National

Exhibition grounds instead of staying in the hospital downtown. It's so they can make money selling food from the concession stands. I can see the posters from my bed, garish shout outs for Tiny Tom doughnuts, deep-fried Mars bars, Bubba's butterfly chips. It isn't right. And I'm going to expose it. Reporters start to arrive. I can tell they're media because they're ostentatiously checking cellphones and BlackBerries. Some have cameras. I check my microphone and start.

I go from the ICU back to Cancer Ward 2, this time to a private room right opposite the nursing station. The nurses at the desk can look straight into my room and see me. Every part of me is attached to something mechanical. My Hickman line now snakes up to an extra-large IV stand; it looks like the mother of the IV stand I had before. I have an ileostomy bag attached to my abdomen for fecal waste, a catheter for urine, a tube down my throat for oxygen, a tube up my nose for food. My entire body is swollen until the skin puffs up shiny and tight on my arms, legs, and face. I can move my arms only with great difficulty and I cannot move my legs at all.

What I learn later is that a part of my intestine started to perforate (a side effect of the chemo, which thins the intestinal lining), causing waste from inside my intestine to leak into my bloodstream, basically poisoning it and sending me into septic shock. But the nurses and doctors managed to get me a scan and then into surgery in record time, saving my life. The surgeon cut out the damaged part of my intestine and stuck the two ends outside to poke out of my belly, the small end, the fistula, covered with a dressing, the larger end, the stoma, covered with an ileostomy bag, for the waste to drain into.

I tell Simon much later, in a wondering tone, "I have no memory at all of that week!"

He answers grimly, "I wish I could forget it."

I had no idea how serious it all was until I read his post from that time:

JUN 22, 2014 9:50 AM

I imagine that many people will have been worrying the past few days due to the lack of new posts, so I wanted to update everyone now that I feel able to. On Tuesday Manjusha required emergency surgery following complications due to the chemo. Manjusha spent 4 days in ICU & her life was very much in the balance for 48hrs. Thanks to the expert medical care she received, Manjusha has made good progress & is now back on the ward. She is currently extremely drowsy due to the painkillers, and it is sure to be several days before she will be able to share her musings with you all.

Thank you all for your amazing support.

I am on saline for hydration, morphine for pain, anti-nausea meds, and sleeping pills. The clocks stop working. I think I hear my mother's voice in the hall talking to the nurse.

"Mom!" I call out. I see that it is five o'clock, which is the time my mother arrives every evening. The nurse comes in. "Where's my mom?" I demand. "It's five o'clock."

She looks at me, puzzled. "It's five o'clock in the morning," she tells me. And then somehow it's three o'clock. Time does not just stop, it goes backwards and the morning often forgets to come. Everything happens in slow motion. Every time I blink, the darkness descends so slowly I think it's someone's arm reaching across me, casting a shadow on my face, and I flinch.

I am desperate to go home. I know about consent to treatment. I know I have autonomy. I have rights. I am convinced they are keeping me here purposely, that the doctors are benefiting financially from trapping me in my hospital bed. Even my trusted friend Homer is in on it. He is paying for his home renovations by keeping me sick. He wants to rig up his second floor so that it can bend and lower itself down to the ground so you can exit the house without troubling to go down the stairs. I can picture his house bending down, like a person bowing gracefully, letting Homer and his wife and their three daughters simply step out of their bedrooms onto the front lawn.

Sunnybrook Hospital is a ship that is bearing me away. Where is Simon? I am being kidnapped. He has to rescue me while we're still on shore, because once we set sail it will be too late. I'm frantic. Where is he? They have already done it once before and yet here I am again. How have they managed to lure me on board again, how stupid and trusting am I? A nurse tries to take my blood pressure and temperature but I refuse to let her. I shake my head stubbornly when she approaches me with her thermometer and blood pressure cuff.

"Please," my mother begs, frantic herself, "just let her do it."

I ignore both of them. I strain to get out of bed, to swing my legs over the side, imagining I could somehow wrestle myself into my wheelchair and push myself out of here, but I can't move my legs even an inch.

I pick up the phone on my bedside table and call 911. I tell the 911 operator I'm at Sunnybrook and need to be rescued right away.

"What?" is all I remember her saying.

I don't have the breath to explain. I have to hang up. Suddenly, I'm surrounded by people, my doctors, more nurses, Simon, my mother, and, improbably, my friend Sharon, who is here to visit.

I look down at her hand gently resting on my swollen fingers and I feel doubt for the first time. What is she doing here, I wonder. She doesn't fit into the whole being-kidnapped-on-a-ship scenario. I frown. My doctor explains to me where I am and I try to take in his words.

"So, I'm not on a ship?"

"You're not on a ship, you're in a hospital."

"A hospital *building?*"

"Yes, a building."

"In Toronto?"

"Yes, in Toronto. It is not a ship. It's not going anywhere. You are not being kidnapped."

But I remember believing that so vividly that it still feels like I was. The time I was taken away by ship, I still think.

I remember that time. They blame my sleeping pills and change the prescription. I apologize. Homer does not mind. "It's not the first time a patient's called 911 on me," he says.

It turns out I never held a press conference either. But I don't find that out until much later when I mention it in passing to Simon.

"What press conference?" he asks.

I eventually come up with a strategy to test if what is happening is real or not. I tell myself to open my eyes. It sounds strange, because of course I think my eyes are open. And then when I open them I find, for instance, that I am not wandering in a post-apocalyptic war zone, but am in my hospital bed, which seems comforting, for a change, in comparison.

In that war zone, everything is dusty and bombed out, people are dashing around trying to keep hidden, scavenging for supplies, for food. Everything is gray. A ragged little girl is lost in the middle of it all; she looks terrified.

"Just open your eyes," I urge her, "this is not really happening." I open my own eyes and find myself in my hospital bed, my hand still outstretched to reach her, my words still echoing in my ears. I had said them out loud.

Another night, I think the world is ending. We are under attack by aliens and we have to escape in fighter jets that keep whizzing by, one after the other, and I keep being unable to flag one down for me and my family. It isn't only me, the whole world is at risk. We are all going to die.

I feel like I now understand, really understand, those parents in family court who think the Children's Aid Society is getting enriched by apprehending their children and placing them in foster care. I think of those claims now sympathetically. Because paranoia is about powerlessness. Even if the choices are all bad, we still need to know we have them. Fear is never completely groundless even as it twists what is real. There *are* forces set on destroying us, only they're not from outer space, but from within our own bodies, assassins traveling up our own bloodstreams.

CHAPTER THIRTEEN

IN THE FACE of the horror I cannot control, I become fixated on one goal, something concrete I can achieve with careful planning. I want a banana Popsicle. I ask the nurse for one the minute she takes out my breathing tube.

"No," she says, "the feeding tube has to come out first, and it can't come out until you show you can eat on your own without choking."

"Eat what?" I ask.

"Like applesauce," she suggests.

"Okay," I say immediately. She leaves and returns with a small plastic container of applesauce with a foil cover you peel off, like one you would put in a child's lunchbox. She has to spoon it into my mouth because I still can't use my arms very well. I immediately gulp down several mouthfuls to prove I can do it and so they take the feeding tube out of my nose.

I ask for the catheter to come out as well because it is really painful, but that ends up meaning they have to put me in diapers, since I can't walk to the toilet, so it is not an improvement. I never think these things through.

Once the feeding tube is out, the hospital nutritionist comes by to offer me a variety of disgusting protein drinks, which I refuse. I am breaking my promise about eating. But that's just too bad, I think. I feel no shame at all even though I never eat another mouthful of applesauce again after those first demonstrative gulps.

"You have to eat," Simon tells me. "No matter what it tastes like."

"You should eat only what's delicious," I intone. I am quoting actress and lifestyle guru Gwyneth Paltrow from one of the magazines a volunteer brought me. Simon is not impressed.

I ask again, during morning rounds, "Now can I have a banana Popsicle?" My hematology team says it is up to the surgical team. The surgical team says ask the hematology team. It's like having divorced parents and not knowing yet who is the soft touch.

June visits and I beg her to find me a Popsicle. She hops up ready to oblige and the next thing I hear is her in the hall asking a nurse brightly, "Excuse me, where do you keep the Popsicles?"

"Noooo," I think, "ix-nay on the opsicle-pay!" I had meant for her to sneak a Popsicle. Finally I nail down someone from the hematology team to say yes, it's okay with them if it's okay with the surgical team. I ask a surgical resident who starts again with "So long as it's okay with hematology," but I stop her mid-sentence. Oh no you don't, don't start this again, and confirm for her that, yes, yes, yes, it is okay with hematology. She hesitates and then says, Fine.

The next day I eagerly await Simon's visit, thrumming with anticipation. But what he brings me are some fancy purple frozen tropical fruit bars because our grocery store does not carry banana Popsicles. I eat one so as not to hurt his feelings, but I'm crushed. Another day he brings what are advertised on the box to be banana Popsicles, but they are creamy, more milk-like, than juice-like. I don't even bother to eat one. I'm disappointed. Simon is unsympathetic. He refuses to search the city for a banana Popsicle.

Then my friend Lisa arrives with one from a convenience store near her Riverdale home—it's exactly what I wanted. It's a neon chemical yellow, it's frosted with white, it's perfect. It's Proust's madeleine, the fleeting taste of which he says calls to life the world of his childhood.

I probably should mention at this point that I don't particularly like Popsicles, or even bananas for that matter. But like that famous madeleine, which apparently is a kind of ordinary cake, not especially delicious at all, a banana Popsicle exceeds the sum of its artificial parts. It tastes of the peaceful boredom of long, hot, sticky summer afternoons when a sweaty bike ride to the tuck shop to get a banana Popsicle was the highlight of the day.

Soon other friends are finding sources for banana Popsicles (typically those grimy stand-alone freezers that sit at the front of convenience stores) and just about every visitor I have hands me a few with great pride and pleasure. I think I may still have them in my basement freezer at home.

I only wanted the one.

CHAPTER FOURTEEN

EVER SINCE the doctors took away my sleeping pills, I'm back to my usual lying awake at 3 a.m. worrying about things. But now my worries are huge and all encompassing: Will I walk? Will I live? No longer merely scabs to peel, hangnails to pick at, a sore tooth my tongue cannot stay away from. No longer small actions I regret, that I used to replay over and over, always with an alternative better ending.

Like the time we're in England for the summer holidays visiting Simon's family. When we check our bags for our flight home, we're told the flight is delayed by twelve hours. Instead of leaving at 9 in the morning, it's going to leave at 9 that night. I quickly grab our bathing suits out of our bags before they disappear down the carousel and we call Simon's dad to come pick us up at Gatwick and take us to Brighton for the day. Everyone's grumbling around us but we're delighted to have one more day. The day is uncharacteristically sunny and warm. We make it to Brighton in good time, have lunch at a Chinese restaurant, buy beach towels in the town, and then walk along the pebbly beach. The water is freezing, and the waves knock us down repeatedly onto the stony floor of the sea, but we're still happy. We continue our walk, aiming for the big pier with its burlap slides and rides and fortune-telling booths and stalls selling Brighton rock.

On the way we pass a trampoline. For ten pounds sterling you can be strapped into a harness and then bounce incredibly high, turning somersaults and flying through the air. Jack has been collecting flyers that were blowing on the beach offering half-price discounts, five pounds off. He gives me two, saying, "Now we can go for free!" I explain it doesn't work like that. We stand and watch for a while. Two young girls are bouncing side by side, their long blond hair blowing in all directions in the wind and they're laughing and laughing. I'm entranced and want Jack and Anna to have a go, but Simon feels there's not enough time if we also want to see the pier.

The pier, though, is disappointing. It takes Jack and Anna forever to decide what rides they want to go on. Anna chooses unwisely and gets nauseous on one that spins a bit too abruptly. We buy the wrong number of tickets, not real-izing that some of the rides require adult accompaniment, so then we have to buy more and we end up spending more than twenty pounds and a bit more time than we should have. It's a rush back to the airport, but we make it just in time, skin sunburned and itchy from the salty sea.

All I can picture, though, is Jack and Anna jumping effortlessly on the trampoline we never let them try. Leaping and laughing, while the sun shines alike on their glowing faces and the glittering sea. I see them flying through the air in my nighttime regrets more clearly than I remember anything else from that trip.

On the first day of grade 4, Jack was starting a new school. "The teacher will probably ask everyone what they did in the summer," I tell him. "Why don't you take in one of your souvenirs from Paris to show? You can talk about what we did there." He likes that idea and chooses his favorite souvenir, a snow globe of a tiny Paris scene with all the monuments crammed close together, the Arc de Triomphe, the Eiffel Tower, Notre Dame. I had thought he would choose his metal model of the Eiffel Tower, not the delicate glass snow globe, but I don't say anything, just wrap the globe in newspaper and put it in his backpack.

When he gets home from school, he's bouncing up and down with excitement. He's had a wonderful day and he loves his new teacher. All through dinner he can't stop talking about all the things they did, and all the things they're going to do, and all the pets in the classroom, fish, lizards, guinea pigs. He wants to head out to the ravine immediately to find snails for the tortoises.

Then, as I pick up his knapsack to take out his lunchbox, I notice it is leaking water. My heart sinks. The glass dome of the snow globe is shattered. Jack bursts into tears, he's inconsolable. I feel even worse because it was my fault for suggesting he take it. What a stupid idea. And they didn't even talk about what they did this summer. He never even took it out of his bag.

After he and Anna have gone to bed, I sit with my teary eyes and my iPad, looking up Paris snow globes on Kijiji. I find dozens, but not the same one. Over the next few weeks Simon helps me research how to make your own snow globe. "It'll be even better now," he tells me. "It'll be more special, because when he looks at it he'll remember how hard you tried to fix it, how much you cared." I'm not convinced, but we buy distilled water, glittering flakes, special glue. We can't find a glass globe but we use an old baby food jar because it fits on the base perfectly. It's still sitting on Jack's bookcase. I don't know if he thinks of it at all, but any time I go into his room I see it and I remember. In the night I close my eyes and I can see the snowflakes swirl all around the arches of Notre Dame Cathedral, even though we went there in the summer.

I hesitate to mention my other big regret: choosing Stanford over Columbia for my journalism master's. Stanford is the better university overall and I was swayed by that fact and the fact that I got a full tuition scholarship there and only a partial one at Columbia. But Columbia has the more renowned journalism program and of course is in the more exciting city. There would have been much more to write about living in New York City than in Palo Alto, California. I wasted almost my entire year at Stanford picturing being at Columbia instead. My regret was real, and sleep-depriving, and enervating. But I know what my readers are likely saying. Really? These are your worst regrets? Breaking a snow globe? Choosing the wrong world-class university?

Fuck you, you *deserve* to have cancer.

CHAPTER FIFTEEN

I DELAY PRESSING my call button for as long as possible, even though I need to have my diaper changed. I've needed it for several hours but I'm trying to hold off because I hate asking too often when the nurses have so many more important things to do. I hate being a pain.

On my bedside tray, I have my usual collection of white Styrofoam cups of water: one rustling with ice, the straw still unbent, its little paper cap still on; the others, half empty and tepid, the straws leaning wearily off to the side. Every time a nurse or orderly comes by, they give me another one. I can't bring myself to take more than a few sips, even though I'm constantly being warned about dehydration and kidney problems, because I pee enough as it is, and I don't want to be the patient they complain about at the nurses' station. Since my room is the closest to the station because of my whole ICU brush with death thing, I can hear most of their conversations.

Say there's a fire, I think, and they have to pick which patients to rescue first, who are they going to go for? The picky, whiny, constantly buzzing because their diaper's the teensiest bit wet ones, or the stoic, uncomplaining, come by only if you have nothing better to do ones?

Exactly.

Babies seem unbothered, untroubled, unruffled by the whole diaper-changing process. I don't understand how this can be. When Jack and Anna were infants, they didn't seem to mind it all. And I didn't even mind doing it. I thought I would. Although I had babysat a lot as a teenager it was never with actual babies, so the first diapers I changed were for my own children. We used cloth ones to be environmentally sound and changed them the second they got wet because they're not as leak proof as disposables. And instead of using those cold diaper wipes, we used cut-up J-Cloths (that got softer and softer after being laundered) dipped into a tub of warm water. Jack, especially, seemed to enjoy it. He would "awoo" delightedly and I would "awoo" right back at him like we were doing backup together on Aretha Franklin's "(You Make Me Feel Like) A Natural Woman."

Finally I can't stand it any longer and press the call button. I hope that young gentle nurse comes—the one who's soft, with both her voice and her hands. But instead, two older nurses show up. They're fun and friendly and chatty (and somehow always work in tandem) and I'm usually happy to see them, just not on diaper duty.

"Come now, honey, turn on your side for me," one directs, while she continues her complaint to the other about some administrative mix-up. "So you know I tell her I didn't get no email about no schedule change, but she say I sent it this morning, but girl how am I supposed to get it this morning when my shift start at seven?"

With a huge effort I turn partially onto my left side and cling to the bed rail with my right hand. I've barely shifted, but it's the best I can do. My body is a dead weight almost beyond my control and even this slight movement takes a lot. My fingers are already slipping off the rails and I don't know how long I can hold on. This is their cue to leave the room immediately in search of supplies.

One comes back with a single wipe. Uses it. Promptly leaves to get something else and I don't see her again for fifteen minutes. Then the second one leaves for a fresh diaper and a clean sheet. By this time, the first nurse is back with the diaper rash cream, which she slaps on quickly; it's very cold. I want to die of embarrassment. I want to stab myself to death with the tiny pair of scissors they have left lying among my flannel sheets. No, wait, I want to stab them first and then myself. I want to wake up and be a judge again, not an overgrown diapered baby.

This whole waiting for the perfect moment to get a diaper change, and then getting it, has taken the entire morning. It's lunchtime now and Simon arrives to take me outside in the wheelchair, an equally daunting production. Simon circles around the ward to find an orderly and asks him to bring me a wheelchair. It takes a while to find a working one. Then I buzz for a nurse to come and unhook me from my IV pump, which means my request has to be made and accomplished between the bags of medications. And it can't be just any nurse, but one who is specially trained regarding IV lines because they have to be cleaned and clamped carefully for fear of infection or blockages.

Then I need two nurses (because one is not strong enough) and the sling to lift me into the wheelchair. The nurses wedge the canvas sling, with its dozen differently colored straps, underneath me and then attach the straps to the winch on the ceiling, carefully matching the colors. The electric winch lifts me up and I sway in the air like a beached whale that has to be returned to the sea. The nurse operating the winch carefully lowers me into the wheelchair, the sling now bunched in hard ridges underneath me. Simon kneels down to unjam the footrests, tucks a pillow behind my back and a shawl around my shoulders, and finally we are off.

Of course this is my cue to pee.

But I don't care. I feel a swell of something that takes me a few moments to identify as happiness. We are leaving the ward. It takes ten minutes to traverse the long hallways, but finally we're outside. The sun is coming out from behind a few clouds. There's a breeze and it smells only like air, nothing else. We bump along through the parking lot, Simon threading me expertly between the cars, because bumpy as it is, it's still smoother than the sidewalk, and then we hit the path by the ravine.

Simon takes me for a little ride first, before we stop to have lunch. The groundhog is at its usual position, edging toward the picnic tables in search of scraps. We pass by the daycare center that never seems to have any children in it.

We go as far as the moose. Years ago, these brightly painted, almost moose-size sculptures were scattered all over the city. But I haven't seen one for a while. This is a sick moose in an ill-fitting blue hospital gown. We visit it every lunch hour. I pet its bandaged leg; it's cool and smooth to my touch.

We retrace our steps down to my favorite bench because it's in the shade. Luckily it's free. There are cigarette butts scattered underneath the No Smoking sign. Simon parks my chair at one end of the bench, facing the ravine and he sits on the bench and faces me. He has sandwiches for us, cheddar cheese, tomato and cucumber; and a can of Coke for me. The breeze is a bit chilly, so he tucks the shawl more carefully around me. We always seem to pick the time when someone's noisily mowing the small patch of lawn behind us.

"What are you thinking?" Simon asks, since it is unusual for me to sit even for a moment without speaking. I bite my lip, and look down at the trees, instead of at him. I know he thinks I'm not ready, but I say it anyway, all in a rush: "I want to go home."

He doesn't answer, just hands me the Tupperware container of chocolate chunk cookies. I eat two, saving my last sip of Coke until I'm finished so the crumbs don't choke me. My throat is thick with longing to go home. We only have about forty-five minutes from the time we left my bed because Simon has to be home when Jack and Anna return from school. Simon puts the containers away and takes me back to the ward.

Homer happens to drop by as we make it to my room. I stay in the wheelchair, Homer sits on the edge of my bed. He congratulates me on my latest biopsy results. He saw from my chart that the second induction chemo worked and the number of leukemic cells in my bone marrow is down to less than 2 percent—which counts as remission.

I don't say anything in response, because I've already taken my results for granted. So the brutal second induction chemo worked and, added bonus, it didn't kill me. Time for a victory lap, but I refuse to do one in a wheelchair.

"That's great you went out," he goes on. "How are you doing?"

"I want to go home," I tell him. Simon has his back to us, putting his Sudoku book and newspaper into his knapsack as he gets ready to leave.

"Are there stairs leading up to your house?" Homer asks.

"Yes," I sigh.

"How many?"

"Maybe half a dozen, cement steps." I try to picture them in my mind.

"Could a ramp be put in?"

"It would be pretty steep," I say doubtfully. Talking about ramps makes it all seem more real than I'm prepared to believe. How long exactly does he expect that I will be in a wheelchair? He makes it sound like it may be months. And there's more.

"Look, even with a ramp, you can't go home until you can at least get from your bed to the wheelchair by yourself," he tells me. "Because you don't have a winch at home and Simon won't be able to lift you."

Simon has turned around now and doesn't say anything, but I can tell he is alarmed at the very prospect. I see the panic in his eyes. I feel huge, unyielding, a sack of cement. Doesn't

he want me at home? Who wouldn't want me at home? I feel
that paranoia again. Is Simon trying to keep me in the hospital? Shouldn't he be just as desperate to have me at home?
I want to be at home right now. Simon and Homer both say
it would be better to go to a rehab hospital first to get mobile
again. I can't bear the thought.

"It would only be for a few weeks," Homer says. But "few
weeks" and "only" do not go together. It seems like a picture
of eternity. I can't go to another institution. Doesn't anyone
understand how unbearable this is? It has been almost three
months in hospital already. I want to go home.

But everyone, except for me, is in agreement, and so the
rehab hospital it is. Now the problem is being well enough to
go there. They won't take me unless I have been fever-free for
forty-eight hours, because fever means infection and they're
not equipped to provide medical treatment, only physio-
therapy. It takes another week to meet that test. Finally,
one Friday, an ambulance is booked to take me to St. John's
Rehab. For some reason, the transfer cannot happen until
after 8 p.m., which is not a great time for me; usually I'm
ready to go to sleep for the night by then. Instead, there is the
bustle to prepare me.

Simon packs up my belongings: clothes, shoes, coat, laptop, iPod, books, snacks, pillows; I have amassed a surprising
amount of clutter. A nurse unhooks my IV lines and caps
them. Two orderlies come in with a stretcher and heave me
onto it to take me to the ambulance, where they strap me in

a bit too tightly. It's still light outside and it feels strange to be driving through the city on a summer evening. I'm feeling motion sickness from lying down and feeling the swerving and the stopping and starting at each red light. Simon is following in our car.

The ward room is two or three times the size of my Sunnybrook room. Its four beds are spaced well apart, so there's enough room for everyone's mobility devices—canes and walkers and wheelchairs. I'm assigned a bed by the far window. It is now almost 10 p.m. I have not had dinner. The nurse says she will try to find me something, but I don't want anything. It is all too much. She returns, carrying a small tray of food in one hand, and wheeling the vital signs monitoring station with the other. She takes my temperature.

"You have a fever," she says, frowning, "38.2."

"I think it's just from the stress, the ambulance, and moving, and everything," I struggle to convince her. "Could you try again in half an hour? I'll probably be fine by then…"

"No," she says. "I'm sorry, but I have to call the ambulance." Before I can even believe this is happening, I'm back on the road, this time in the dark.

We get to the Sunnybrook emerg at around 11 p.m. It has to be the emerg because I'd been discharged, so I no longer have my bed on the ward. I wait there for an hour, strapped tightly to the ambulance stretcher. I ask the medic to loosen the straps a bit. A man waiting near me has incredible body odor. I feel like I'm going to throw up. I ask to be moved closer to the entrance so I can get some fresh air. A doctor finally admits me, and I'm taken back up to the cancer ward.

The doctor, a stressed, yet kind, young woman, gets into

an argument with a nurse right at my bedside. It turns out what I thought was a long time was actually a short time; the doctor had skipped some bureaucratic steps to get me back into the cancer ward relatively quickly, and the nurse is not pleased about it. The doctor is frustrated and explains to the nurse as patiently as she can that she didn't want to leave me hanging around emerg any longer.

"Fine, write it up," she finally tells the nurse in exasperation. She puts in a requisition for a few scans to check the source of the infection. They're scheduled for midnight that night and end up being inconclusive. It's not clear what kind of infection I have, or if I have one at all. I no longer have a fever. But now it's Saturday, and nothing can be done until the weekend is over. And because it's the weekend, no doctors or physiotherapists come by.

I'm not very good at waiting. When I'm waiting for something, I cannot do, or think, of anything else. All day Saturday and Sunday I just wait; I don't pick up any of my books; I don't watch the next episode of *Downton Abbey*; I don't chat on the phone; I just wait, as tightly wound as the clock I'm staring at. Hang on, maybe this means I'm actually very good at waiting?

My family would disagree. I used to drive everyone crazy when we went for dim sum at one of those cavernous places where women push around carts of steaming bamboo baskets. Simon, Jack, and Anna would sit patiently waiting for the carts to come by our table, chatting and playing the "what's missing?" game where Simon removes something from the tabletop, and Jack and Anna have to guess what it is.

"Close your eyes, close your eyes, close your eyes," he

would intone, while whisking away, say, Jack's chopstick holder, and hiding it in his lap. Jack and Anna would sit with their eyes scrunched tight, trying their best not to peek. Meanwhile, I was too distracted to participate. I'd be bobbing up from my chair, squinting across the room, trying to see what was coming.

"Mummy's water glass?"

"Nope."

"Anna's napkin?"

"Nope."

"The bottle of—"

"The har gow and sui mai cart is heading this way!" I'd interject excitedly, "Here it comes, here it comes…. Ohhh, wait. No, it turned, I can't believe it!" When I finally couldn't take it anymore, I'd leap up, run down the aisle with our little form to be stamped, and retrieve the dumplings myself.

On Monday morning the ambulance takes me to the rehab hospital again. This time I don't have a fever, and I'm allowed to stay. I don't manage to score a bed by the window; instead, I'm assigned the one by the door. I also don't get diapers because they've decided I need to work on using the bathroom. They start by trying to teach me to get in and out of bed by myself. To get out, I first have to find the control pad on the side of my bed (sometimes obscured by the mattress and sheets and blankets), and press the button that lowers the whole bed closer to the floor. Then I have to press the button that tilts the bed to put me in an upright sitting position. If the bed rail is up, I can't see the control pad and have to do it by touch. The bed contorts wildly before I get it right.

Once I have managed to both lower and tilt the bed, I have to cling to the rail and sit unsupported, and swing my legs over the side. I have to use my hands to grab my pajamas and yank my legs over the side, as they don't move easily on their own. Finally, I have to feel with my feet for my slippers, which often have been kicked under the bed by the nurses' comings and goings. If I can't reach them, I give up, and go barefoot.

It's at this point that I have to have a nurse help me into the wheelchair. I can get the wheelchair to the bathroom by myself, but the door is too heavy for me to slide shut, so the nurse has to do that. If I don't have a nurse, I leave it open—I have no modesty anymore. A nurse has to help me onto the toilet. Then she goes away to do something else. I wish she would stay with me because I'm done in a minute, but she has many other things she needs to do. So I have to press the buzzer in the bathroom and wait for a nurse to return to help me back into the wheelchair and then back into bed. Eventually, I can manage in the bathroom by myself, but I still need help getting into bed. One evening, I wait forty-five minutes in my wheelchair, watching the light fade from the large windows at the end of the room, until a nurse has time to help me back into bed.

Once in bed, it's very difficult to settle into a comfortable position, because I can't move very well. So a nurse teaches me how to use the T-bar that is dangling over my bed. I have to grab it with both hands and use it to inch my whole body up higher on the bed so I'm in the right position. The first time I do it, I pull all the muscles around my abdomen and for the next month it feels like there is a tight band wrapped around my torso, squeezing me, not painfully, but uncomfortably. It takes so long to dissipate, and leaves so gradually, that I don't even register when it's finally gone.

While I'm game to go through all the steps to use the toilet to pee, I'm resistant when it comes to changing my ileostomy bag. Since the surgery a month ago, the nurses at Sunnybrook have always changed it. But here they want me to learn how to deal with it myself. It's hard because I've been in such denial about it that the first time it leaks, I panic and call for a nurse, thinking some vital fluid is trickling out of me. The nurse actually laughs, because I'm being so silly about the equivalent of a poopy diaper. I eventually meet them halfway and learn how to empty it myself, which has to be done every couple of hours. But every week, the bag itself has to be peeled off me and a new one stuck on. This I cannot do. I cannot even watch while they do it, cleaning and measuring my stoma, cutting a hole in the flange to fit it, clicking the bag into place once the flange is stuck on. I avert my eyes or shut them altogether. I can't bear thinking about the two ends of my intestine poking out, never mind looking at them, and really never mind touching them.

To the nurses, though, it's no big deal. One comments on what a perfect job my surgeon did.

"Stoma perfect," she pronounces, "like rose. Like right from textbook."

She even brings over a nurse-in-training to take a look at how perfect it is. When I ask why the bag fills so quickly, she explains, "Stoma working, working, working." She snaps her fingers to indicate just how efficiently it is working. "Not like bowel, waiting for socially acceptable time, this needs to be emptied every hour or two, all day, even night."

I can't face it, and yet it's hard to think of anything else. It's hard to take any pleasure in eating, when you can see so clearly and immediately what all you have eaten turns into.

In the *Little House on the Prairie* books, which I continue to reread to this day, Laura Ingalls Wilder describes all aspects of pioneer life in painstaking—and, frankly, often tedious— detail. There is a whole chapter on Pa building a door for the stable, for example, or an addition to their claim shanty. All aspects that is, except for a critical one. There is never any mention of Pa building an outhouse, not in the Big Woods, not on Plum Creek, and not by Silver Lake. I used to wonder how they managed when the girls were babies, for instance, or when they were confined to their house for the whole of that Hard Winter.

When Ramona, in another of my favorite series, asks her kindergarten teacher how Mike Mulligan managed to go to the bathroom when he couldn't leave his steam shovel all day, the teacher answers by saying it's not mentioned because it's not important. The class is skeptical; of course going to the bathroom is important, and the teacher knows it. Why else was the location of the bathroom the first thing she showed them on their first day of school?

In the hospital, certainly, it's all anyone seems to talk about. Especially during mealtimes. My lifting the cover off my dinner plate is the cue for the nurse to question my neighbor in minute detail about the frequency and quality of her bowel movements. The elderly woman in the bed opposite me refuses to use her buzzer to call the nurse. Instead, she yells out "Pee!" when she has to go to the bathroom, which is a dozen times during the day and through the night. Her daughter, a beautiful, stylishly dressed twenty-something-year-old, explains, over and over again, as does the one nurse who can speak Cantonese, "Press the button and a nurse will help you get to the bathroom!"

Five minutes later I hear the familiar yell, "Pee! Pee!"

CHAPTER SIXTEEN

THE WOMAN who has the bed next to me is very friendly, gushingly so, at first. "You're so beautiful!" she says one morning, as her mother pushes her wheelchair past where I am sitting in the chair by my bed. "Your skin just glows!" She even praises my cheekbones, which I guess are thrown into relief by my bald head.

Then her mother pipes in, clearly also wanting to compliment me somehow, "And your son is so tall!"

They have not yet seen Jack. They are referring to Simon, who is six foot three. At least their flattery makes sense now. For someone who has a forty-six-year-old son, I do look pretty good.

Her friendliness ends abruptly when I ask her to turn off her overhead light one night. It's almost 10 o'clock. I've been fretting since 8:30 about when would be a reasonable time to bring up the issue of the light. A nurse carefully doles out one sleeping pill to me each night. It takes about thirty minutes to take effect. If I take it while the light is still shining brightly it won't work, and it will be wasted because I've found if I don't fall asleep in that first half hour, the night is shot. I'm tossing and turning, figuratively that is, as I can move only with great difficulty. I sleep on my back, in almost a sitting position. I long for the time I can lie flat, curled cozily on my side, one hand tucked under my pillow. It's now 9:45. We each have control over an overhead light and a reading light. Because the curtains separating us don't reach the ceiling, when one overhead light is on it's pretty much as bright as if all of them were on.

I rehearse the words in my mind: Would you mind turning off your overhead light, I'd like to go to sleep? Sorry to be a pain (insert friendly self-deprecatory laugh here) but could you turn off that light? Do you think…The nurse arrives with my sleeping pill. I take the easy way out, scrunch up my face in a pained expression, point to the light, and whisper to the nurse, "Could you ask…" The nurse immediately goes over to the next bed.

"Time to turn the light off, other patients need to sleep."

"But I'm reading," the woman protests. "I can't go to sleep this early."

The nurse is curt. "Use your reading light."

"It's not strong enough, my eyes…" The nurse just stands there. "I can't read by it…" Her protests dwindle. "…not one word." Finally she repeatedly yanks the pull cord and the light clicks, first brighter, then brighter still, then finally off. But I'm tense now, imagining that compliments from her are no longer going to be flowing my way, and I don't fall asleep for hours.

The food is worse than at the hospital. I'm actually nostalgic for Sunnybrook's tortellini and grilled cheese, which now seem like the height of culinary perfection. Here the bread at breakfast is like a piece of wood. I think it was toasted outside the city somewhere and then trucked in. I crumble two or three bites off the crust and eat it with the shrink-wrapped orange cheese.

Simon brings sandwiches for lunch as usual. The grounds are lush and extensive. The nuns (whose place this was before it became a rehab hospital) were good gardeners. We go to the place where the flowerbeds and benches are arranged around a large stone fountain. We watch several chipmunks chase one another around the edges, sometimes balancing precariously on the slippery gray brink for a drink. They manage not to fall in, though it's close. Simon always brings nuts. He gets to the point where a chipmunk will climb up his leg to perch on his knee for a snack.

I never used to want to be anyone other than myself, and now I constantly look at people and wish I were them. I see a young man in the reception area one day, in a well-fitting dress shirt, holding a briefcase. He immediately leaps up to give me his seat when he sees me approaching with my walker, but I thank him and wave him off, and as I pass I have an intense longing to be him, which I have never felt before. I imagine he is there for a job interview. I've thought about him a lot since. I wish I were a young, handsome man, just finishing school, eagerly attending job interviews.

I think that whenever I see anyone who looks young and

healthy, especially if they have nice hair. Frankly, I think that even when I see the chipmunks. I'd even rather be a rodent, I muse, if I could be a healthy one.

Simon and I go to a seminar in the ward's common room about how to stay safe at home. The presenter goes over slide after slide, all about the dangers of falling down. Falling, apparently, is the first step to a slow, excruciating death and must be protected against at all costs. Get dressed sitting down. Iron sitting down. Wash dishes sitting down. Be careful not to trip over the vacuum cleaner cord. "I never realized all these things were so dangerous!" I whisper to Simon.

"You don't have to worry," he reassures me.

"Because I'm careful?"

"No, because you never do housework."

Good point, I think. I never ironed or vacuumed even when I was healthy, so there's no way on earth I'm going to start now that I'm recovering from cancer. I remember a silk shirt I bought when I was in law school. It was dark purple, and shiny and soft, and fit me perfectly. But, once it went through the washing machine, it was a crinkled mess, and since I don't iron, I never wore it again. I don't remember what happened to it.

When Simon's mother came to visit us from England to help out after Jack and Anna were born, she asked me where the vacuum cleaner was and I couldn't tell her. I had no idea where we kept it, and we had lived in that house for more than a year by that time. She had to wait until Simon got home.

I have never fallen, never worried about falling, and now I'm scared. The woman farthest from me in my ward room fell down some steps on a train trip through the Netherlands last summer. That's how she ended up here. I have pieced together her story by overhearing her phone conversations with friends. It sounded like one of those times when you've reached your destination, but there's an announcement telling you to remain seated until the train has come to a complete stop; but no one ever pays attention because they're too busy gathering their belongings from the pockets of the seats in front of them, or from the overhead compartments, and anyway the train is going *so* slowly. Then there was a sudden jerk as it came to a final halt. She fell down some steps, broke her hip, ended up in a European hospital at huge expense, and then at home in rehab for months. Whatever you do, do not fall down.

I had already decided I was never going to go downhill skiing again. It was something we had recently started to do as a family. Simon was an experienced skier, and Jack and Anna picked it up quickly. I was terrible and terrified, but willing to try. No longer. Not a big sacrifice, I thought, because I do need to be more careful now, and I certainly don't want to end up in hospital again.

But the presentation slides are not warning about the dangers of skiing. They are about the dangers of stairs and socks, and those fringes on the edges of carpets. It seems either nothing is dangerous, or everything is. I may as well keep skiing.

Still, I'm more bored than scared. Simon is past bored. There is still an hour to go. How many more variations on the theme of not falling down could there possibly be? We're trapped in a far corner. I'm in my wheelchair and there is an obstacle course's worth of wheelchairs and walkers between us and the door. I don't care.

"I have to go the bathroom," I stage-whisper apologetically to the woman beside me. Finally the primacy of bathroom functions works in my favor. She shuffles back a bit, Simon grabs the handles of my wheelchair, and we make our escape, albeit very, very slowly.

Later, I overhear the doctor taking a group of residents through the ward. "Leukemia used to be a death sentence," he tells them. "Most people died." They scuttle after him right past the foot of my bed.

"Now it's the reverse, most people survive."

Hooray, I think.

"Pee! Pee!" the old lady yells.

CHAPTER SEVENTEEN

I WANTED TO ATTEND my stem cell drive on July 13, but I'm not in good enough shape to leave the rehab hospital. Kate and June give me a detailed account of it. Not only did they find all the rectangular tables they needed, but they found the donors. They were hoping to attract at least one hundred people to be swabbed, and in the end, 170 turned up, mostly young men, the most desired demographic because they have more stem-cell-rich blood than women. There were almost as many volunteers as there were potential donors. Dozens of friends and colleagues donated their time and provided food. There was lunch for the volunteers, many of whom stayed the whole day rather than just for their shift, and snacks for the donors. Even TV celebrities turned up—Sukhi and Jinder, contestants on *The Amazing Race Canada*. And an eleven-year-old girl, Cierra, who also was hoping to find a donor, and who eventually did find one, made an appearance with her parents to thank everyone.

Then, on July 19, I learn that several potential matches have been found for me, 10/10 and 9/10. In the end they can't confirm any of the 10/10 donors. I'm guessing it's because the people are unavailable or unreachable for various reasons. But they are able to confirm one of the 9/10 matches, and the transplant is a go. Since it takes several weeks to process a cheek swab, the timing means the donor must have been from an existing registry, not from any of my swabbing events.

The million-dollar question during my last interview with Alisa for the radio documentary is "How did you feel when you found out you had a match?" Unfortunately, I don't have a dramatic answer, because it all happened so quickly. I'm focused on learning to walk again. I still have a third round of chemo to face, before I can even be considered a candidate for a stem cell transplant. I, who worry so much about everything, have not even had a second to wonder if a match would be found, before it was. The unlikeliest step of all in this journey, incredibly, ended up seeming like the easiest.

"But that's bad!" I say, much later, when Simon and I are lingering at the breakfast table, after Jack and Anna have left for school. My tea is cold, but I'm still taking small sips of it to delay going upstairs to my computer to write. Simon's reading the *Globe*. "I was thinking all this time that finding a match would be the climax of the whole book. But it won't write like that. It's a nothing moment. Not exciting. Not dramatic. Why!?" He looks up and thinks for a moment.

"I guess we had other things to worry about." He's right, but I still feel like I've failed my narrative.

One time that first year when my friend Alison is visiting me in hospital, we get on the subject of our happiest days. "My happiest day this year was in January," I tell her. "It was the one sunny day we had in Mexico and we went snorkeling and saw sea turtles. Jack and I saw an eagle ray. We ate tacos at a café right on the beach. We watched pelicans diving in the water. It was so great."

"My happiest day this year," she says, "is when I found out you got a match." Her response moves me deeply, but at the same time, it indicts me. That's the answer I should have given.

In the movies, when the hero (usually some tough athlete or cop) is learning to walk again, the thrilling moment is at the parallel bars when he drags himself along, grunting and sweating, to swelling music in the background. And I was looking forward to that. But I actually manage okay with the bars. My ability to walk while holding onto something comes surprisingly quickly. It's releasing the bars that's hard.

"Let go of your walker," my physiotherapist, Caroline, instructs me, a few weeks into my stay in rehab. I do, and she moves it out of the way. She has accompanied me back to my room after our session, and we're standing in the area between the door and my bed. She pushes my tray table out of the way as well. She turns back to me. I haven't moved because I'm afraid of falling. She raises her hand in front of her. She's holding a small green bean bag, which I hadn't noticed before. She drops it on the floor and it lands almost exactly between us.

"See if you can pick it up," she tells me. I grimace. She must know I can't bend over, that I still have to use a plastic stick with a grip on the end to put my pants and socks on.

She says, "Go as close as you can." I inch my feet farther apart to give myself better balance, making sure to avoid stepping on the laces of my right moccasin slipper which, as usual, have come undone. I should cut them off, I think, they're really just for show. Without realizing it, I have bent all the way down and when my surprised fingers make contact with the bean bag I instinctively close them around it and pick it up. I straighten, smiling for real now.

"I did it!" I tell her, as if she hasn't witnessed this miracle for herself. Then she tells me something even more miraculous.

"You can probably go home on the weekend," she says. It's Wednesday now.

"How about tomorrow?" I ask.

"Well," she hesitates, "the doctor has to sign the discharge papers and he's already left for the day."

"Can't he sign them tomorrow?" I ask. She agrees.

"He starts his rounds about 9:30. If you catch him right then, you could leave in the morning."

I wake up hours early the next morning, I'm so afraid of missing the doctor on his one trip through the ward. To my relief, I'm able to get the right papers signed by the right time. But, as Simon is about to wheel me out of my room, a visitor drops by. It's a former colleague. It's sweet of her to come. I haven't seen her in years. I don't want to be rude, but I cannot spend one more second in that room. I take the delicate spray of white and purple orchids she has brought me and hold the little pot on top of the pillow and plastic shopping bag of paperwork I already have in my lap. I suggest we chat as we head down to the parking lot, so Simon can go ahead and get the van. I listen distractedly to her anecdote about how her daughter did an internship at this very rehab hospital.

"What a coincidence," I murmur, all the while keeping my eyes peeled for Simon and our minivan. There it is. I can't wait a single second more. I thank her for coming, and wrestle myself into my seat while Simon folds up the wheelchair and puts it in the back. I'm free.

CHAPTER EIGHTEEN

"REMEMBER ME?" The doctor is wearing a mask but I can tell by her eyes that she's smiling.

I squint up at her from my wheelchair. At first she doesn't look familiar at all, and then, "Oh," I say slowly, "wait, from the cab that time?"

I'm back in Sunnybrook. I had managed to do the week of consolidation chemo from home, but when a follow-up appointment found me feverish and too tired to even sit up while waiting for the doctor, I was readmitted. I had barely enough time at home to scrape a groove in the dining room hardwood with my walker. Now I've been wheeled down to have a biopsy, because of fears I have a fungal infection in my lungs. Two doctors come into the examination room and I realize I know one of them.

We had met while standing shivering in a long line for a cab at the airport one snowy evening last January. I had started to chat with her because she seemed friendly and the line was just inching along. We discovered we lived fairly close to each other, so I proposed sharing a cab. It turned out we had both been in Ottawa for conferences, mine judicial, hers medical. We had a lot to talk about in the cab because her children were about the same age as mine, and also in French immersion. I never expected that I would see her again, much less have her be the one threading a painful scope down my throat, while I coughed and spluttered helplessly.

As my eyes tear up and I gag on the scope, she is reassuring: "Almost done. You're doing so well." And even when she takes the scope out and says apologetically that she has to do it again because she couldn't manage to get a proper sample the first time, she says it so kindly that I almost don't mind.

"The good news is that Jack and Anna are okay." These are Simon's first words to me. I'm alarmed rather than reassured. He had correctly anticipated that my first question for him that day was going to be "How was the camping trip?" But I had not anticipated his response; not at all. We've been going camping for a week every summer with the same group of families since Jack and Anna were three years old. This year Jack and Anna went without us, taken instead by Sharon, Paul, Cole, and Noah. Since they don't have a car and were going to rent one, I had insisted they borrow our minivan.

"What happened?"

"Sharon was brushing a spider off her lap and her hand hit the steering wheel. She drove off the highway and crashed the van."

I can't think of anything to say.

"No one was hurt, but the car's totaled."

Apparently, the front end crumpled, and every window shattered. I see Jack and Anna later that same day, and they seem unbothered. Jack's eye is slightly red where it had been hit by some bits of glass. Anna had been protected by her glasses, one of the lenses of which was slightly chipped by the flying glass. It was over so quickly, they didn't have time to panic, they tell me. Before they knew it, they were sitting by the side of the road joking and chatting with Cole and Noah, while waiting for the other camping friends to collect them and bring them home.

Since I hear about it only when it's all safely over, I don't have time to panic either. But it makes me realize that I had been assuming I was immune, at least temporarily, from other tragedies. I can't be in the hospital being treated for leukemia *and* have a child die in a car accident. Right? *Right?* I hadn't realized it until this moment, but, since my diagnosis, I had stopped worrying about Simon and the children, and now I have to start again, even though the only lasting impact was the one on our car.

The spring when Jack and Anna were two and a half, we went to an international children's theater festival to see a play called *Rabbit in the Moon*. It started with a woman who passed out little slips of paper and pencils and asked us to write down our deepest fears. She then collected them to take them to the moon, but before she did so, she asked some people in the audience to read their fears aloud.

"I'm afraid my son will die," the woman next to me said. Her son, maybe six years old, was sitting beside her at the time.

I was astonished. Doesn't she know you can't speak these things out loud? Who knows who is listening, and what power over life and death they possess. I don't remember what worry I wrote down, but I know it wasn't a real one. I thought then that there were things you could do, or not do, to protect yourself. I thought there were rules. Worry all you like, but never speak your worries out loud, was one of them. I did not know then, that voicing or not voicing, worrying or not worrying, makes no difference at all.

When the play ended, the ushers beckoned to Jack and Anna to lead everyone out, and off they went, hand in hand, as directed, through the curtain. I was so surprised that they went trustingly, without protest, when usually they were shy, that I remained still sitting until the curtain fluttered closed behind them. And only then did I leap to my feet, to scramble through the other audience members, so I could follow them out before they got too far ahead.

Why do I ever let them out of my sight? Come to that, why did I go through all the paperwork to get them British passports, of all things? Why do I worry so much, yet aid and abet them to go so far away? They disappeared once for a few seconds, and each subsequent disappearance will be longer and longer until, poof, they'll be gone.

My first roommate this time around is an old woman, gentle, with a faint British accent. Her husband is gentle as well, with a faint German accent. Once in the evening when she hears me weeping with despair (as I am wont to do), she calls out, "Would you like my husband's hand to squeeze?"

It makes me smile, even as I decline. Her children and grandchildren seem similarly sweet and innocent. I overhear her commenting to her daughter once about how quiet it is on the ward.

"Barely any visitors around today," she says.

"Oh, well, you know, you're at the far end of the hospital," her daughter replies. I picture fed-up visitors stopping, worn out, at the bedside of just any random patient, because it's closer than the one they have actually come to the hospital to see.

"When you can walk, you can go home," the physiotherapist encourages her cheerfully every day.

"I will walk *when* I get home," she responds, uncheered and unencouraged. "They fixed one thing and ruined another. They didn't start the radiation soon enough. I could walk when I came in."

"So that means we have to do physio," the therapist counters brightly, undeterred. "Let's do ten minutes. Try lifting your right leg, come on now, easy, peasy, lemon squeezy! It's a matter of functionality—"

"I don't need you to lecture me, I'm seventy-nine years old."

"Either you want to participate or not." The physiotherapist who started out speaking to her with over-the-top enthusiasm like you would use with a toddler eventually becomes testy and starts to talk tersely about how she is a professional with years of experience, and the woman needs to listen to her for fuck's sake. She doesn't exactly say for fuck's sake, but it is clearly implied; in any event, her tone is a far cry from the lemon-squeezy she started with.

"I'm going," the woman's husband says, his voice shaking, as he gets up to leave the room. "I'm too mad to stay."

"Don't you want to stay and see what we're doing?" the physiotherapist asks. "All you do is push her in her chair. That won't make her better."

"Do you think she'll ever have strength in her legs?" he asks.

"The doctor will reassess. We should have a family meeting."

"No." He goes. The physiotherapist sighs in exasperation.

"Don't you look at my husband that way!" the woman says quickly.

"I didn't look at your husband in any way. If I wanted to say something I would say it."

The standoff was messy, but the solution is elegant. In an impressive "make it someone else's problem" move, the upshot is that since she came to Sunnybrook from another hospital, really they are the ones with the authority to send her home, and so she's sent back to the first hospital.

She is replaced by another older woman with two middle-aged daughters, whom I can't tell apart. They dress in similarly shapeless skirts and blouses and even wear the exact same running shoes. They spend night and day arguing loudly with the doctors and nurses about what treatment their mother should be getting. They speak so harshly that I don't even recognize their language as Spanish (which I have always thought of as so musical) until a Spanish-speaking nurse converses with them. They are always pushing for more tests to be done, and then redone. They commandeer a wheelchair as an extra place to sit, since there are two of them, even though wheelchairs are scarce on the ward.

When they push into my space, I push back. I am not giving up an inch without a fight, I decide.

I wake one morning to find they have moved their mother's bed, so it's right up against the curtain between her bed and mine, to make more room for themselves on the other side. But when nurses need to access the woman from the curtain side, which is several times a day, there's no room for them to stand, so they have to stand in my space, which means I can't get out of bed as my IV stand is on that side.

I speak to my nurse about it, and she makes them put the bed back to where it was, which makes them hate me forever. There are a lot of raised voices and angry accusations that it isn't fair. They think my side of the room is larger to begin with, thoughts they share in detail with every nurse and every visitor.

I win that battle, but lose the ongoing one about the bathroom. If they hear me even start to stir out of bed, their mother hobbles to the bathroom as fast as her stiff legs can take her, so she can get there first. I'm convinced she doesn't even have to go—that it's just payback.

I mentally give my own ending to Sartre's famous line: Hell is other people...in the hospital bed next to yours.

The sisters are either both there, or one is there and the other is available on speaker phone, around the clock, barraging the doctors with requests for more and more tests, while the doctors with infinite kindness and patience explain that their mother's pain is muscular, not indicative of a return of the cancer, and what she really needs is to be in a rehab hospital, not a cancer ward. I wait to see who will break first. It seems like she is winning because I keep hearing them set discharge dates that come and go and there she'd still be. But one miraculous day, Sunnybrook flat out refuses to redo some scans, saying the old ones are perfectly fine, and actually discharges her to a rehab hospital.

I am discharged August 29, after I prove I can go 48 hours without a fever, only to be readmitted five days later because I'm sleeping 24 hours a day. I can't even manage to get up for meals. They suspect it's the $10,000-per-month fungal medication that's to blame. I had been put on it as a precautionary measure, even though the lung biopsy was not definitive about whether I actually had a fungal infection.

When I'm admitted this time around, no beds are available in the cancer ward, so I end up in some general ward with three other women, all much older. The woman across from me complains about everything at the top of her voice, starting with the delivery of her breakfast tray at eight o'clock in the morning.

"Three orange juices! Who can drink three orange juices?! This is outrageous! I want the supervisor! I want to call and make a complaint! This is ridiculous! Who can drink *three* orange juices?"

"You don't have to drink them," I say. "Throw them away." Who cares? I think. Why does it matter? I don't have the energy or breath to speak very loudly, plus the tears are starting. She hears me, but just glares and keeps going. She buzzes constantly for nurses and yells more complaints if they take more than five minutes to arrive. I try to ignore her but I can't. A woman visiting her mother in the bed next to mine looks at me with great sympathy, and then goes over to the complaining woman.

"Do you think you could not shout?" she asks her gently. "There are other patients here. They're really sick. They can't take this noise." The woman looks at her blankly and keeps up her angry complaints.

I finally make it back to the cancer ward, and the roommate I have the day before I'm discharged is the best roommate I've had to date. It's too bad it's for the shortest time. We bond immediately, because it turns out she is exactly my age, forty-seven. We share the injustice of being too young to be so sick, surrounded as we are by patients in their seventies and eighties, patients whose grandchildren are older than our children are.

She and her husband are soft spoken with some kind of eastern European accent. He has longish, wavy hair and looks artistic. Her daughter is sixteen and spends most of the day at the hospital with them. Her cancer seems to be in an advanced state; she can't get out of bed, and her only drug is morphine, which she self-administers through an IV drip. She comments admiringly on how I can manage to get to and from our bathroom by myself, and I remember to feel lucky.

I go home on September 7, and the next hospital visit is not mine, but Simon's. He's admitted overnight to have his thyroid gland removed, because they found pre-cancerous cells. I'm overwhelmed. Could this really be happening to us?

Could I get leukemia, the children get into a car accident, and Simon get thyroid cancer (the distinction that it is "pre"-cancerous is lost on me at the time), all in the same summer? Apparently we can, and apparently we can just roll with it. In fact, the whole house has been revolving around me for so long that Jack's only reaction on hearing that Simon has to go to the hospital overnight is "But who will take care of Mummy?"

In my journal, Simon, in his minuscule handwriting, carefully notes down the schedule of my medications:

Before breakfast: voricanazole, Pantaloc

With breakfast: magnesium, potassium, Marvelon

Before dinner: voricanazole

With dinner: magnesium, postassium

Bedtime: zopiclone, hydromorphone

On the same page, he also notes which of the above prescriptions need refilling, and when the nurses last changed my ileostomy bag and the dressing for my Hickman line.

On the very next page are my notes from the same time period:

Kiawah Island, South Carolina

Aruba, Eagle beach—best

Turks & Caicos, Smith's reef—great snorkeling!

Secrets Aura Cozumel, adults only, swim up to room

Iberostar Grand Rose Hall, Jamaica, great reviews, lobster!

CHAPTER NINETEEN

ON THE OUTSIDE of Princess Margaret Hospital, there is a banner that declares, in capital letters more than a foot high: WE CAN CURE CANCER IN OUR LIFETIME. I had taken that less as a fundraising slogan and more like a sacred covenant. Our lifetime means my lifetime—means my actual life.

Inside, Simon and I are sitting, listening to the transplant team list all the ways, and all the times, the transplant could be fatal to me:

> You could die right at the time of the transplant itself if it does not "take" (that is, if the donor stem cells do not set up shop in your bone marrow and start producing immune cells), because we will have eradicated your own immune system through intensive chemo and radiation, so you will end up with no immune system at all.

You could die shortly thereafter, even if the transplant does take, of acute graft-versus-host disease, if the new immune system (the graft) fatally attacks your organs (the host), which it will perceive as invaders.

You could die subsequently, of chronic graft-versus-host disease, if the new immune system decides to attack your organs later.

You could die at any point of an infection, since we will be suppressing your new immune system so that it does not attack your organs, which means it is not as available to attack infections.

Swimming in fresh water, eating unpasteurized cheese or sushi, exposure to direct sunlight or large crowds could also kill you, because all of the afore-mentioned, besides being among your favorite activities, carry increased risks of infection.

On the bright side, you could survive any of the above and live out your life as an invalid. You could possibly return to work sometime between one to two years post-transplant and never.

Sign here and here and here to acknowledge you are fully aware of all the ways this transplant, which is meant to save you, could actually terminate your life prematurely, or leave you a fragile shell of your former self. Because really, what do you have to lose?

You have a greater chance of dying if you don't have the transplant, because the leukemia could come back and you probably wouldn't survive another round of induction chemo. (Remember what happened last time!)

It occurs to me that the Hippocratic oath, rather than the "First do no harm" of popular belief, should actually be "You can't say we didn't warn you."

Yet, without discussing it, without researching it, without thinking about it even for a minute, I sign and sign and sign. Even as tears are trickling down my face, I sign, because it is clear this is my best chance for a cure. That is what I hear, even though those are not the words they ever use.

What I am drawing on is not my medical knowledge, which is zero, but my knowledge as the mother of a preteen girl. I know my subtext. When Anna is past the point of no return, regarding hunger or sleep, I can tell, because that's when she refuses all offers of food and resists going to bed. When she is hostile and moody, and pushing me away, she is actually asking me to demonstrate my unconditional love for her. It took me a long time to hear her meaning, rather than her words, or her tone.

And my father thought there would be no use for an English literature degree.

When Anna was seven years old, Simon, returning from a trip to the doctor's with her, reported that she had cried after getting her flu shot. Before I could commiserate, he added, "She cried because it didn't hurt, not because it did." I stopped, confused. He explained that she cried because she had been dreading getting the shot so much that when she found out it wasn't painful after all, she regretted the time she had wasted dreading it.

Even her meltdowns at the age of two were similar. After a tantrum one morning, over an issue whose origin I can't even remember, she insisted I shower again. I had showered just half an hour earlier, so I refused to give in to what I considered to be another irrational demand, on the principle that, as with terrorists, you should never negotiate with toddlers. I regret that now.

It wasn't an irrational demand. It was a desperate desire to start the day afresh, because she regretted the time she had wasted having a tantrum. Her wish to turn back time in the hope of a new beginning, a happy outcome, wasn't childish at all, but an elemental human desire. What was childish, and therefore so moving, was her belief that it was possible.

I wish I had acquiesced, back when I possessed the power to turn back time itself; the power to be Superman, reversing the earth's orbit, and bringing the dead back to life. The day will start anew. No one will get upset. No one will be diagnosed with cancer. All I had to do was step back into the shower.

Simon takes me to Princess Margaret Hospital for the first of two full days of tests to prepare for the stem cell transplant. It ends up being nonstop poking and prodding from 7:30 a.m. to 4:30 p.m. Blood work, lung function tests, CT and MUGA (heart) scans, and the one I've learned to fear because I've now had it three times, a bone marrow biopsy. At least that day's doctor reassures me she is fairly confident the leukemia is still gone, because my blood work results are good. But worse than the many needles is her rundown of the horrific possible side effects of the transplant, such as infections, diabetes, loss of my sense of taste, secondary cancers, and repeated hospitalizations to deal with graft-versus-host issues.

"Eat all your favorite foods now!" she says, in what I feel is an inappropriately cheerful tone.

"Do you think I could go back to work by the spring?" I ask. I think I'm being sufficiently cautious and realistic, but she responds with an unequivocal "No."

"Twelve to eighteen months post-transplant would be realistic," she says, and I'm so busy calculating that instead of early 2015 this could mean as late as the end of 2016 that I almost miss her adding, "Some people are never able to return to work full-time."

When that sinks in, my eyes fill with tears. Simon squeezes my hand and his eyes are red-rimmed as well. Being a permanent invalid seems even worse than dying to me.

In an attempt to alleviate the situation, she quickly adds, "I have a patient who is twenty years post-transplant and doing great." I wonder, is that an anecdote or a promise? I ask when I can get my ileostomy reversed (so my intestines are safely back inside, where they belong) and she gives me the same depressing time frame of twelve to eighteen months after the transplant.

I keep going. "How soon before I can travel, do you think?" I'm thinking of the cruise we had booked for my parents' fiftieth wedding anniversary in a month's time. We had to cancel it, of course, but I'm trying to calculate how long before we can rebook it. I'm also thinking of my optimistic list of recommended vacation spots, collected variously from friends and TripAdvisor reviews.

"You have to take things one day at a time," she explains. "Try not to plan out the future."

This goes against every grain of my being; but I guess I'm going to have to work on it, otherwise I'll face constant disappointment. Also, I'll become paralyzed with depression if I think of normalcy as being a year and a half away. I have to think about how to make the hour I'm in as happy, and bearable, as possible.

"At least she didn't mention any risk of dying this time," I say to Simon as we leave, trying to extract something positive out of the meeting.

"That's because, now it's going ahead, there's no point talking about that," he answers.

I had actually thought it was because the risk had magically disappeared. I feel my old optimistic self inside me like one of those Weeble toys I used to have, those tiny egg-shaped dolls that immediately bob up when you push them over. "Weebles wobble but they don't fall down!" was the accompanying commercial jingle.

When will you ever learn, I say to my inner Weeble.

It ignores me.

The last check is by the hospital dentist. They want to make sure there is absolutely no problem, because even a tooth infection could become fatal in the aftermath of a stem cell transplant, when you have no immune system. The dentist is cheerful and kind and pleased to report that my teeth and gums are fine.

"Book a follow-up sixty days post-transplant," he tells me as he's walking out the door.

"Wait, what?"

He pauses and looks back at me expectantly.

"Uh, nothing, that's fine, I'll do that." He smiles again and leaves.

What I had wanted to do was confirm with him that his casually asking me to book an appointment two months after my transplant was actually him assuming—no, *promising*—that I would be alive at that point. I decide that would be pushing it, but I'm elated nonetheless and can't wait to share the news with Simon.

"He asked me to book my next appointment for the end of December," I announce to Simon, when I rejoin him in the waiting area. "*December*, that means he expects that this will all be fine, right? Because otherwise why book an appointment for *after* the transplant? You wouldn't do that for nothing, right?" I'm doubtful again, though, when I consider a friend's visit right before my transplant. Despite his busy work and family life, he drove all the way from Boston to Toronto (a round trip of eighteen hours) just for me. At the time, I was delighted to see him, but now I'm thinking, maybe he made all that effort because he thought it might be his last chance to see me.

This is getting too confusing. It would be easier and, frankly, more scientific to read tea leaves or scattered chicken bones.

Simon takes me to Toronto General Hospital on October 21 to get a Hickman line put in again. The doctors had taken it out in that brief period I had between the consolidation chemo and the transplant. Now I need the line for more chemo and for the stem cells. Because it hadn't hurt the first time (other than my feelings from that doctor ignoring me), I consider booking tickets to the musical *Wicked* in the evening following the appointment, because Anna really wants to see it. But it's a good thing I don't, as the procedure is agonizing this time around.

The surgeon freezes one side of my neck and then starts inserting the tube into the vein on the right side of my chest, where the tube had gone in before, only to be foiled because the vein is blocked. He jabs repeatedly, but is unsuccessful getting through. He periodically increases the freezing because I'm trembling with the pain. Just when I think I can't bear it any longer, he announces that he's sorry, but he has to give up on the right side and repeat the whole procedure on the left side of my chest.

I now have the added worry of blocked veins, and so I ask him fearfully if he has to do something to address that.

He laughs and says no, that your body uses other smaller veins around the blockage instead, "so your head won't explode."

It takes me a second before I feel reassured, because you don't like a doctor to ever, ever, use the words "head" and "explode" about you, even if they are separated by the word "won't."

The pain is awful. Not only at the surgical site, but all through my neck and upper back. My head aches, my teeth are throbbing, and it hurts to swallow. I sleep on and off all day, and I look a bit scary with my neck bandaged on both sides, tubes dangling off one bandage and a pink stain all around (that I first think is blood, but then realize is the pink solution they cleaned the area with before the surgery). I am self-medicating with the hydromorphone tablets I have left over from my most recent stay at Sunnybrook. I'm assuming that is okay.

My surgeon on this go-round was charming, referred to me constantly as "dear," and talked me through every step. But it was so painful, during and after, that it made me think fondly of the doctor who did it the first time around without speaking to me, because that time, it didn't hurt at all. I feel like I should take back my complaint.

Homer and Vivian visit me before my transplant, bearing multiple containers of takeout dim sum. I tell them about how I read that a stem cell transplant costs $500,000 and I ask at what point will they stop offering me all these expensive treatments? So far, I seem to be getting the absolute best the Canadian medical system has to offer.

Homer says there is an actual formula Western countries use. They will spend up to $100,000 to prolong your life for a year. On that calculation, a $500,000 stem cell transplant is a good deal, because the expectation is that it will give me, not just five years, but the rest of my natural life.

I'm constantly calculating in my mind, shuffling the years, the odds. I'm forty-seven now. If I can live for fourteen more years that would take me to sixty-one, which I believe is the earliest date at which I can retire with a reduced pension. That's important, because then Simon and the children will be financially secure. Fourteen years mean Jack and Anna will be twenty-five, which isn't bad. They'll be finished university by then.

"Don't you ever think about you dying?" I ask Simon.

"Only when you bring it up," he says.

I've never been to Las Vegas, never gambled anywhere, but I keep thinking of my future as something someone is offering me as a bet. Would I take fourteen years, if it were offered to me right now, as a sure thing? Absolutely, I would. But then, when I'm feeling energetic and have had a good doctor's appointment, I wonder, would that be selling myself short? What if I would have lived twenty more years otherwise? Twenty-three years would take me to seventy. Jack and Anna would be thirty-four years old. They could be married, and even have children by then. Imagine, I could dance at their weddings, maybe even officiate at them. I could hold a grandchild, maybe even babysit one.

I mention this in passing to my family doctor when I see her next, and she says, "Twenty years? Why only twenty years? Shoot for thirty!"

I am taken aback at the very thought. I hadn't dared to go there. Thirty years would take me to seventy-seven. Thirty-five years would take me to eighty-two, which is pretty much the life expectancy for a healthy woman my age in Canada. I read about seventy-year-olds going for heroic treatments, searching for organ donors, and I think, really? I would take seventy on a silver platter right now. I don't know why I always picture it like that, on a silver platter, like a lavishly presented gift. Maybe because it's something I would take gratefully, without uttering a word of wistful complaint. It's the certainty I crave, more than the actual number, when I picture making that deal, with whoever it is that is authorized to make deals like these. I would sign over a potentially longer life in exchange for the certainty of a set number of years. In my low moments, I think, Hell, I'd take five good years (on a silver platter).

I'm busily firing off all these numbers at Simon one day, as if they were just that, numbers, when I notice he has tears in his eyes. I'm so consumed by the numbers and the calculations that I've lost sight of what they represent. It's like I've traveled so far from reality, I can only think about it clinically, not realizing that after the five years, or ten years, that I'm willing to make a deal for, I'll be gone. Simon won't have a wife. Jack and Anna won't have a mother. It's a loss I'm trying to guess the start of, not realizing that when it starts, it doesn't end. My life might have a tidy number of years left, but my absence will go on for the rest of their lives. My voice trails off.

Stop talking, I think. You're so selfish. Are you happy now? You've finally made Simon cry. No one is waiting to make a deal with you. This is not a game show. Who am I kidding anyway? TV and radio game shows (like *Beat the Bank*) always make me so tense. Should the contestants keep what they have, or risk it all and go for something more? They might end up with nothing. It's only money, and not even mine, just some stranger's on the radio, and I still can't handle the stress and the disappointment, the clanging bell of the empty vault. It's a good thing I'm not asked to play it for real with my actual life.

CHAPTER TWENTY

"WOW, THIS IS AMAZING!" my friend Nancy gushes. She's popped in on her way to work, at a law firm a block away from Princess Margaret Hospital. "What an improvement!" She starts lining my windowsill with box after box of designer skin care products over my protests that she doesn't have to bring gifts every time she visits. Her own skin is perfect.

I have a private room this time; in fact, it's more like a suite, with a private shower and even a small annex with my own exercise bike. My door is heavy and blocks all noise from the hall. Not only do I not have a roommate, two days go by before I lay eyes on a single other patient. Even the nurses' station is quiet, no bustle or intercom announcements. The only IV alarm I ever hear is my own, and when it beeps and I press for a nurse, one arrives instantly. There is no waiting for nurses here.

The kitchen in the ward has a fridge full of treats for the

patients: Coke, ginger ale, ice cream. Even Popsicles, *banana* Popsicles. Right in the ward.

Things must really be serious now.

The door is heavy, not to block noise, but to block germs. Whenever I open it, the special ventilation system creates a negative pressure so that air cannot travel from the room into the hallway, minimizing the spread of infection.

The reason I have my own full bathroom is so I can shower the required four times a day, because the chemo I'll receive makes your perspiration toxic. It causes skin rashes unless it's constantly washed away.

Every patient is secluded and even the kitchen is locked. You can access it only through a nurse because of fears of infection. There are complicated rules about bringing food from home and where it's allowed to go. They go over it umpteen times but my mother and I still have no idea which part is forbidden. Is it that food from outside has to go straight to the kitchen and can't go to my room first, or is it the other way around?

The windows to the left of my bed face west over the city. I look out on the row of shabby Victorian houses along McCaul Street. I can just make out the first couple of restaurants on Baldwin Street. I can see the University of Toronto, and depending on how I position my chair, I can even see part of Lake Ontario. To pass the time, my mother gazes out the window and gives me a running commentary.

"Oh, it's starting to rain," she announces, when the umbrellas come out. "I never see anyone come in or out of those houses," she adds. "Who lives there?"

I cannot summon up the curiosity to care. The people on

the street seem irrelevant to me. I feel as far away from them as the stars are from me. They're going to work, to school, to restaurants, out there in one of my favorite parts of the city; but my Toronto has been reduced to a single room. I feel so distant that I never close the blinds when I change. I feel that invisible. Sometimes I don't even bother to close the blinds at bedtime, because the sun is that negligible November sun that makes the city seem grayer in daylight than at night. At least the night has contrast; it has edges; it is definite.

I will first get high-intensity doses of chemo and radiation, and then the transplant, on what is called Day Zero on the little highlighted calendar taped to the wall at the foot of my bed. I will be released once my white blood cell count reaches 0.5, which hopefully will be by the end of November, or specifically, Day 25. I stare at the calendar night and day, willing the days to pass.

The ward is so quiet, I hear only the white noise of the air ventilation system, which is loud but unspecific, so I soon don't hear it at all. It muffles all conversation, and everything seems muted. There is only one sound, a low thrumming, and only one smell, a cross between a medicine and a cleaning product. It makes me queasy.

I was really worried when we first arrived because I threw up two times on the way to the hospital, making Simon pull over for an emergency stop by the side of the road. Not only was that embarrassing, but I thought I had caught some stomach bug on this most important of days. But when I first meet the specialist on the ward, he explains that it is a result of the pain from the Hickman line procedure. He orders some codeine for me and I feel better as soon as I take it.

"It hurts a lot more when they have to go in on the left side," he explains, "because the veins are lower down, which means more probing." He is tall and boyishly handsome and speaks in kind, measured tones. He is hugely popular with the patients and nurses alike. It makes me feel much better knowing the reason for the pain. He doesn't act like he's in a hurry to continue his rounds, so I ask about my other concerns.

"I was worried," I tell him, "at my first appointment, when they said the transplant might not take. I got the impression, I guess, that...does that mean that's the end?"

He shakes his head and smiles.

"We have a plan for that," he says. "We purposely harvest more stem cells from the donor than we think we'll need. So we can do a second transplant, if we need to."

"What about graft-versus-host disease?" I keep going. "What do you do if that happens?"

"Graft-versus-host generally doesn't occur until after discharge. That's why, when you leave here, you'll have to keep coming back in twice a week for about two months to get checked. It's actually good to have some graft-versus-host effect. We infer from that that the new stem cells are strong. Because, if they're attacking you, your organs, they're probably also attacking any residual leukemia cells in your body."

"I thought I was in remission!" I say, alarmed at the thought of "residual leukemia" lurking in my blood. He shakes his head.

"They never know if they got one hundred percent of the cancer cells. But we've found that patients who experience graft-versus-host disease have better long-term outcomes."

When he expresses it as "outcomes," it feels cool and detached, not like my life or my death, just different outcomes, and I do not have any inclination to weep, even at the new thought of leftover leukemia cells lurking in the hidden bends of my bloodstream.

The next day, though, I am down again, when he tells me I will have the Hickman line in my chest for six to nine months after my discharge, because I may continue to need it for blood transfusions. I do a quick count on my fingers and am devastated to find that this means I may miss a second summer of swimming. But I decide to keep those same fingers crossed. A cautiously optimistic average of seven months takes me to the end of June, so I may still get July and August in the water.

When I spellcheck my CaringBridge post about my swimming calculations, it highlights my first name as an error and suggests "minutiae" instead.

When my chemo finishes, I go down to the radiation department for two full-body radiation sessions: forty-five minutes in the morning and another forty-five minutes in the afternoon. Lining me up exactly takes almost as much time as the radiation sessions themselves. I have the marks inked on various parts of my body from the measurement session I had before my admission to hospital. But it still takes a long time for the technicians to be satisfied that everything lines up. They even tell me where to direct my gaze.

I am allowed to blink, but otherwise I have to remain

perfectly still while the radio plays some indie rock station. Even though I know you can't feel radiation, I imagine that I can. An invisible laser attack on my body, killing every last remaining bit of my immune system. I imagine being hollowed out and then filled with a stranger's stem cells. Because you can't see stem cells, they seem like nothing and like everything at the same time.

All through this ordeal, none of the medication has made me as nauseous as this radiation does (or perhaps it is the cumulative effect of all the treatment). Nausea and despair taste the same. I can't tell which of the two I'm feeling. The day after the radiation, I throw up several times and am unable to eat anything. My nurse, who comes in later that evening with my sleeping pills, sees me lying in bed with tears streaming down my face.

"Are you crying because you miss your children?" she asks sympathetically. "You could Skype them."

I try to smile. I don't reveal to her that I'm not thinking about them at all. I'm crying just because I'm sick of being sick.

It is 2 p.m., October 28, 2014. Day Zero. The day I get my stem cell transfusion. More than 2,000 kilometers away, 150 teachers in Dallas, Texas, blow me a kiss. It's at the request of my friend Peter, who is conducting a workshop at an educational conference there that same hour.

The afternoon I get the stem cells seems celebratory and buoyant. This is what I've been waiting for; this is the final step. I feel elated. My mother is there. Simon was there but has left because it's time to get Jack and Anna from school. The nursing supervisor is there with all her paperwork, checking that everything is in order. She stays during the whole infusion, which doesn't take long. It's just another small bag I get by IV, seemingly no different from all the bags I've had before.

"It's basically a battle of good versus evil."

When I ask my friend Bharati, a geneticist, to explain my stem cell transplant to me, this is how she begins. This is more like it! I thought for sure she would tell me something I wouldn't understand, but this I get. Not science, but a saga. My cancer cells are Death Eaters, waves of Orcs from Mordor, dragon teeth sown on fertile soil, multiplying Hydra heads. The stem cells are Harry Potter, Frodo and Elven armies, Greek gods, and Marvel Universe superheroes. But they don't just do battle for your life, they are the first seed of your life itself, the magic bean that can grow not only into a giant beanstalk, but into anything.

You start life as a single stem cell. When one sperm fertilizes one egg, to create you, the first thing you are is one cell, and that cell is a stem cell.

Cells grow by dividing. So that first cell divides and becomes two, and then those two become four, and those four become eight, and so on. At some point, very early on, the stem cells get a signal that tells them what kind of cells to become: skin, liver, brain, lungs, etc. Once they get that signal to specialize, there is no turning back. Once a liver cell, always a liver cell. By the time you're an adult, you have stem cells remaining in only three places: your bone marrow; your circulating blood; and your umbilical cord blood (if you happen to have banked it).

The job of the stem cells in your bone marrow is to make all your blood cells: the red blood cells, which carry oxygen to all the parts of your body; the platelets, which aid in clotting so you don't bleed to death if you're cut; and the white blood cells, which fight infection. Some of your body's cells live for days, some longer; but none live forever, they are constantly dying and being replaced.

The way stem cells divide is different from the way other cells divide. One liver cell divides to become two liver cells, but a stem cell can divide to make a mother stem cell and a daughter stem cell. The daughter stem cell then gets a signal to become a particular type of blood cell: red, white, or platelet. But the mother stem cell can go on to divide into another mother and a daughter and so on. Thus they can replicate themselves and make blood cells at the same time. All the blood in your body is constantly passing through your bone marrow, which is how the new blood cells join the flow, and some stem cells are carried along for the ride. Your stem cells make 300 billion blood cells every day.

The quality control required to keep this all going is so mind boggling that instead of wondering why something went wrong for me, I'm actually wondering why something doesn't go wrong every day, for every single person on earth.

The error is so tiny at first. Each white blood cell, like every cell in your body, contains twenty-three pairs of chromosomes, which is where all your genetic material is stored. Sometimes a bit of one chromosome will break off and join another chromosome, resulting in genes combining that don't normally combine, causing a genetic mutation. Sometimes these mutations are harmless and the cell dies. And sometimes, like in my case, they are not.

In my leukemia, the particular pieces of chromosomes that broke off and recombined, 4 with 11, and 7 with 10, created a type of genetic mutation with superpowers. And their superpowers are so amazing I have to admire them, really: They are harder to kill than my other white blood cells, resistant even to most types of chemotherapy; they replicate faster; and they survive longer. I'd been wondering why they would be so foolish as to kill their host, but there is nothing to wonder at, because it doesn't happen immediately, it happens generations of cells later. And just like humans devouring the earth, they don't care about that distant future.

As for my other white blood cells, whose job is to fight invaders, were they asleep at the switch? Did they fail me in some way? To be fair, it wasn't really their fault. They couldn't recognize the invaders at first, because they came from within, camouflaged as friends, so they weren't identified as enemies. When my white blood cells finally did recognize them, it was too late. They were outnumbered.

So, in an attempt to save me, they had to be sacrificed and replaced by a donor's stem cells. A donor's stem cells have two big things going for them: They are a close match, but not an exact match, which means they will be able to recognize the invaders, which my cells could not; and they are stronger than my own stem cells were.

The donor is anonymous, but I try to pick up clues about who he or she might be. I get the impression that the bag is not frozen, but fresh, which makes me speculate that this could mean it was from somewhere close so they could get the stem cells quickly.

It is one small bag, which means, I think, that the donation is "juicy," a term I heard to describe blood that is rich in stem cells. Sometimes it takes several bags before you get enough stem cells. But if it is a small bag, it means the donor was likely young and male because they are the most likely to have stem-cell-rich blood.

So I'm guessing it is a young man of South Asian origin living somewhere in or near Toronto. Simon's guess is that it is a young man from Germany because of its large registry. I'm told I can contact the donor a year post-transplant (if he or she agrees). Why a year? I guess to make sure the transplant is successful; you wouldn't want to get to know someone only to learn later that they didn't make it.

It turns out that a few rooms down from me is the sister of someone I know. After my transplant, I knock at her door, dragging my IV stand behind me, to introduce myself and say hello. She is sitting up in bed with her laptop. A case of plastic water bottles is on the floor by her bed, the cellophane wrapping ripped open. A couple of the bottles are on her bedside tray and one is in her hands as we speak.

"I'm so thirsty!" she tells me. "That's good," I say enviously, "they keep telling me to drink, and I'm not thirsty at all." I'm constantly being lectured about how I have to show I can drink at least 2.5 liters of water a day before I can be released, because otherwise dehydration will land me right back in the hospital. I tell her I just had my transplant.

"What was it like?" she asks.

"It was just like getting anything through the IV, like a blood transfusion. It was just one bag, it just took a few hours, and I didn't feel anything."

It seems like it should be a bigger deal, that I should have a more dramatic story to tell. She seems simultaneously relieved and disbelieving that it was such a non-event. Much later, I mention to a friend in passing, "I wonder how she's doing? You know, she had her transplant the week right after me. Her room was two down from mine, isn't that a coincidence?"

There is a beat of silence and then a hushed "Didn't you hear? She died. A few months ago, I think." I am shocked and saddened. I later learn she was readmitted to hospital one week after her discharge, with acute graft-versus-host disease. The stem cells attacked all her organs, and she died a month later.

I didn't know then that the seemingly simple transplant would knock me out. Or, more accurately, I didn't pay attention to their dire list of potential side effects: skin rashes, mouth sores, nausea, and feeling like you have knives in your throat. Because what is the point of paying too close attention to risks you have to take? I was scared and just hoped I wouldn't get everything so badly. But I do. For a full two weeks after I receive the stem cell infusion, I cannot put anything in my mouth. I do not eat one bite of food, take one sip of water, or brush my teeth. I throw up into a blue plastic basin that I clutch at all times. I get my liquids, nutrients, morphine, and anti-nausea medication by IV drip. It is a huge effort to get out of bed and take the required four showers a day. I sometimes skip one, or even two.

My fingernails and toenails all turn black. I'm down to ninety pounds. My mother is anxious. I don't want any of her food anymore. I don't want to talk. I don't want to do anything. She fidgets by my bedside, rearranging things unnecessarily. I don't even have the energy to be irritated, as she moves my Styrofoam cup an inch closer to me.

She's used to leaping to my defense, even when I would rather she didn't. We were walking home from the bus stop one evening when I was eight years old, when a little boy ran by us and yelled "Paki!" at me. My mother was furious. I begged her not to do anything, but she told me to go on home and she marched after that boy right to his doorstep where she gave his mother a lecture on civility. When my brother graduated from university and was living on his own in an apartment in Waterloo, she called him one evening and heard him groaning, "I…can't…come…to…the…phone… please…leave…a…." followed by a beep. Not realizing it was his answering machine (even when she called right back and got the same message), she called her friend, whose son, Milind, also lived in Waterloo, and then she called 911. When Harish came home that evening, he first saw Milind in his lobby—"Boy are you in trouble! Call your mom!"—and then he saw the firefighters in his apartment. But she is helpless now, and it is killing her. Her baby is in trouble, and there are no bullies to berate, no firefighters to call. She can't even comfort me with food. There is nothing she can do.

CHAPTER TWENTY-ONE

I WAKE ONE MORNING to see a nurse sitting in the chair by my bed. She has cartoon kittens chasing each other all over her capacious nursing smock. I look carefully to see how many different colors they come in before the pattern repeats.

"I've been here all night," she tells me, "because you're not supposed to be walking around the ward and you went to the nurses' station at midnight." I look away from the kittens and frown with concentration, but I don't remember doing that.

"You were perfectly polite," she reassures me, even though it hasn't occurred to me that I would be otherwise, even in a delusional state.

"You asked if it was morning, because you needed to make eggs for Jack and Anna. I brought you back to your room and you came with me no problem. But I had to stay to watch that you didn't get up again."

A social worker comes by and gives me a pamphlet for teens dealing with a parent who has cancer. I give it to Simon, but I think it is too much for Jack and Anna because it mentions things like "Many people with cancer survive," and somehow I don't think it's in their minds that I might not survive, and I don't want to put it there. Even though, of course, it's all that's on my mind.

I chat with a student nurse about outcomes one afternoon, when she's changing my sheets, and she says a stem cell transplant gives you ten years on average. All I can think about is that ten years only takes me to fifty-seven (twenty years younger than my dad is right now, and he seems young and healthy to me, still driving us places, still fixing things at home and at their cottage).

"That is ridiculous," says Kate firmly, when she calls from Ottawa to check in on me, and I tell her anxiously about the ten-year average. "That's not true at all. The outcomes are so much better than that. She doesn't know what she's talking about. She shouldn't have even been discussing this with you!"

A spiritual advisor drops by frequently as well. I was suspicious that the visit would be religious, but it isn't at all; it isn't even especially spiritual. She is just a very kind woman with whom I can chat about my worries.

When I'm able to resume my laps around the ward, towing my IV pole, I stop to read the little copper plates screwed into the frames of the paintings that line the walls. This is a mistake. I had been admiring particular pictures as I kept passing them in my endless circles, but it is only now I discover that my two favorite pictures are donations from the families of patients who did not make it. That this could be so had not occurred to me.

I'd been thinking of what painting I would donate, but I certainly won't be doing it if I don't make it. I don't think I could be that grateful. One of my favorites is a restful painting of a stream through a wood, donated by the wife of a man who died at age forty-four. The other is a sketch of the Tasmanian devil (from the Roadrunner cartoons), by a patient who died at age eighteen. The sketch is bold and detailed, but what really moves me is that it is framed in little stickers, which seems more a thing a child would do, rather than a young man.

I wake up with the worst sore mouth I have ever experienced. It's impossible to swallow, and all I do is sleep away the long morning into the afternoon. By then the doctor adjusts my medications, adding an IV steroid and increasing my morphine, so I'm able to talk and swallow without pain and can even welcome the music therapist who comes by every other day. She usually speaks softly to me about how I'm doing, and plays vaguely recognizable, soothing melodies on her keyboard (like *Minuet in G*). But today she's bustling with extra energy.

"You know what we should do?" she asks, and then answers before I can respond, "We should write a song together."

"Oh, I can't do that," I tell her. "I used to play the piano, but I've forgotten everything. Plus, I'm pretty sure I'm tone deaf."

"I'll write the music," she says. "You tell me what you want it to be like. Maybe it can be for your kids." I perk up at that.

"Can it be a song that they can play?" I ask. "Maybe that we can all play together? We did that last year, with Christmas carols. I played the piano. Jack played the guitar. And Anna played the violin. Simon played the triangle. Could we have different parts like that?"

"Yes!" She is enthusiastic. "What kind of melody?"

"Like a folk song," I tell her with, "with a kind of waltz-ing beat."

"How about if we switch the instruments around so it can be for cello or guitar?" she asks. I had told her that Jack plays both, so I like that idea a lot. She tries out a couple of melodies for me to approve, and even though she describes this as us writing a song "together," really, my only contribution is to think of a title. I want it to be beautiful and meaningful, and so settle on a phrase from my favorite e.e. cummings's poem, "I carry your heart."

I immediately have second thoughts, because even though it's a beautiful poem, the line sounds nothing like a title. You can't imagine anyone ever saying, "Hey, can you play 'I carry your heart' one more time?" Oh well. She returns a few days later with all the parts written out. I'm thinking maybe we could play it for my parents' wedding anniversary party, which was supposed to be this December but is now postponed along with all our trips.

The music therapist and the doctor are playing for the opening of the glass garden in the hospital courtyard on Monday at 2 p.m. I have asked if I can go, but it depends on my blood counts. Right now I'm restricted to the ward until the risk of infection passes because my white blood cell counts are low. The flowers in the garden look like the ones from Disney's *Alice in Wonderland*. You expect them to break out in song any minute. They are large blown-glass flowers, in blocks of red, yellow, purple, and pink. They're bright and childlike, and they give me a lift every time I see them. I can look at them for half an hour as if they were a TV show. Time moves in different ways now. The years are flying by (death is imminent as opposed to being hidden in a future haze), but an hour can shimmer like something solid you can touch, like an oversized glass flower.

I remember some author describing how he feels he overuses the word "just," so when he finishes writing, he goes back and takes out all the "justs." It makes me aware that I overuse the word "actually." I think it's because I live so completely in an imagined world, I feel the need to distinguish the times when I am forced to acknowledge that something is "actually" happening. Sometimes my imagined life as it should be coincides with life as it is, but I notice even the slightest deviation when it doesn't.

Let go of the life you planned, wisely counsels so-and-so, and live the one that's waiting for you. But how can I let go of the life I planned, when it is a film unspooling in my head in constant counterpoint to my dreary reality? It was hardest at the beginning. I would lie in my hospital bed and think, Now we should be at Laura's house playing the board game Apples to Apples. Now Simon and I should be watching *Angels in America* in the Distillery District. Now we should all be in London watching the stage production of *The Curious Incident of the Dog in the Night-Time*. Now we should be in Amsterdam lining up outside Anne Frank's secret annex. Now we should be bicycling past fields of gladioli on our way to the Dutch coast. I see them swaying in the salty summer breeze even as I am staring at the static glass flowers in the hospital courtyard, which now seem weirdly purple and red under gray Toronto skies.

A chart is taped to my bathroom door. I'm supposed to write down exactly how much I drink each day, and exactly how much I expel. The drinking part is not too difficult. The little juice cups that come with my meals list exactly how many milliliters they contain. The Styrofoam cups of water each hold half a liter. Yogurt, ice cream, and Popsicles all count. I round up generously, because I'm trying desperately to get to my 2.5-liter goal. I even count the swallows of water I take with each pill.

The expelling part is harder. There is a white plastic container with measurements marked on it that fits over the toilet—I'm supposed to pee into it first before dumping it into the toilet so I can keep track. I do it even though it's a pain, especially in the night when I'm half asleep, to stumble from the bathroom to my night table for a pen, and then back to the bathroom door without getting tangled up in the cords of my IV pole.

What I refuse to do, however, is measure the output from my ileostomy bag. It's simply too gross. I don't want to even look at it, much less measure it, dump it out, and then clean the container. There are limits, and I've reached mine. What I do is try to estimate an amount and write it down every time I empty the bag. It's random, but the nurses end up complimenting me.

"I don't think I've ever seen where the input and output is exactly the same!" one of them exclaims. I grimace, guilty but unrepentant. I never make my 2.5-liter-a-day goal, but I'm discharged according to schedule anyway, because of my fervent promises to meet the goal when I get home.

I'm lying, of course.

CHAPTER TWENTY-TWO

"YOU HAD the perfect excuse to get out of it." Homer can't believe I'm planning to go to Anna's winter concert. "You just had a stem cell transplant!"

I've been home for seven days. I'm weaker than I ever remember being. The first time Simon hands me a glass of water, I almost drop it. I am so unprepared for the weight of the smooth, clear tumbler, after all those Styrofoam cups at the hospital. I don't have the strength to turn on my iPod or to clip my fingernails. One doctor advises against going to the concert because it's winter and flu season; people will be sick. Another doctor says it will be okay, tells me to wear a mask, and try to stay back from the crowd, and adds, "You can't not live your life."

I always keep asking until I get the answer I want.

It's my first venture out in months. It's snowing. I bundle up in sweatpants and a fleece jacket under my winter coat.

I have my cancer scarf wrapped around my still-bald head and a face mask pinched over my nose and mouth. I shuffle slowly down the church aisle, gripping Simon's hand tightly. It is either too hot or too cold, depending on where we are in the church.

It's crowded and bright, and noisy and animated. Parents are greeting each other loudly over the bustle; blocking the aisles with their chatting, hugging, and catching up. Occasionally a chorister scurries by in a black tunic, white shirt, and red bow, long hair carefully tied back. Everyone looks so beautiful: small children in puffy coats; women in lipstick, sparkly blouses, and elegantly tapered pants. I forgot how pretty people can be. We see a friend, but she mimes having a bad cold, and hurries past us without stopping, fearful of infecting me.

We slide into a pew in the middle of the church and are settling in when Simon notices a rear balcony that seems unoccupied. We find the stairs and make our way up, to find only a half dozen people there, including a photographer. We edge by his tripod and sit in the front row of the balcony. The church is long and narrow and we are far from the choir, but I can see Anna as long as I perch on the edge of my seat so the wooden railing doesn't block my view of the front row where Anna is stationed. It's a good thing we moved up here, because two girls throw up on stage, at two different times, right in the middle of the concert, necessitating long interruptions of mopping and toweling.

I end up in Sunnybrook emerg a few nights later, with an infection. They put me in a special waiting room this time because I have no immune system, and then send me home with antibiotics. Next, I get a painful rash on my neck and arms, and start on steroids. It's too much. Simon and I buy lunch at Druxy's in the lobby of the hospital while we wait to pick up this latest prescription. I start crying into my grilled cheese and barbecue chips.

"What's the matter?" Simon asks gently, handing me a napkin.

"What do you mean, what's the matter? I have graft-versus-host disease!" I sniffle.

"They were expecting this," he reminds me. "It's a good sign. It means the stem cells are working." All I can think is, We've come for so many appointments, surrounded by so many patients, and I'm the only one who ever seems to be crying.

The steroids do clear up the rash instantly, but they also give me that steroid moon face, like it wasn't already hard enough to look in the mirror. The tiny steroid pills are on top of the twenty or so pills a day I'm already taking—to suppress my new immune system, to ward off infections, to build up my body's depleted vitamins and minerals, to combat nausea, to relieve pain. Some of the medications serve to combat the side effects of the other medications. I even have a pill that makes it easier to swallow the other pills.

There are also IV infusions I must get for months. A home care nurse comes by to hook me up to bags of magnesium, saline, and anti-fungal medication, for five hours every day. For a few weeks, the doctors add an extra infusion of an anti-viral medication; this one in a portable IV pump, in a bag I have to carry with me, at all times. I keep forgetting I have it, and get up from the table or sofa or bed, only to have it tug me back, like a hand yanking me by the neck of my sweatshirt.

I have to go to the hospital twice a week (every Monday and Thursday morning) for blood work, so the doctors can review counts of this, and levels of that. They make changes to my medications, at almost every visit. It is a finely calibrated balancing act: adding and subtracting drugs, increasing and reducing dosages. The appointments start at 8 a.m. and usually end at noon. But one day, the clinic is especially crowded, and I have to wait into the afternoon.

It's another world. The morning people look shaky and skinny. Many are still bald and attached to IV pumps like mine. The afternoon people are the mythical people I had been told about. They would look ordinary to anyone else, but that is exactly what makes them unicorns to me. They have survived their stem cell transplants. I overhear one woman (thick curly hair! bright pink shoes!) mention that she is eleven years post-transplant. I desperately want that to be me, and even more desperately fear it never will be.

At every visit, I have to fill out a DART questionnaire (Distress Assessment & Response Tool). The basic version is straight-forward, but every once in a while I get the long version, which stumps me with questions like "Are you able to complete household tasks such as vacuuming?" I mentally chew on my pencil while I think of how to respond (mentally, not actually, because I am now germaphobic and I don't know where the pencil has been). Simon reads over my shoulder and I can hear him cluck his tongue. I know what's he's thinking, and I try to defend my affirmative answer.

"It's asking if I'm *able* to vacuum," I point out. "It's not asking if I *do* vacuum." The rest of the questions are easier, but the circles I carefully shade in, ranking my levels of depression and anxiety on a scale of one to ten, get me a referral to a hospital social worker.

I sit in her office, mopping my tears with the crumpled tissues I have in my pockets, Simon at my side, as he is for all of my hospital appointments. She asks if I'm feeling suicidal. "No," I say. "I'm pretty sure I'm not." I look up "suicidal thoughts" later, and then I'm sure I'm not. They're defined as thoughts about how to kill oneself, which can range from a detailed plan to a "fleeting consideration." I am below even fleeting consideration. Something more passive than that. Like idly wondering where Simon put the Percocets I didn't use, and how many are left. Like musing that maybe death would be better, if I don't get better. But despair alternates with anger, and they don't have a circle to fill in for that.

If you asked me right at the time of my diagnosis who my model for a sick person is, I would have said the saintly Beth in *Little Women*, who goes sweetly and uncomplainingly into that good night, thinking only of others, right to the very end. Because isn't that what everyone assumes? Fat people are jolly. Disabled people are brave. Dying people are saints. Sadly, it turns out I am not Beth. I am the first Mrs. Rochester, the madwoman in the attic, in *Jane Eyre*. I want to rage and bite and rend and claw and stab. I don't want to suffer in accepting silence. I want to set fire to my house, and then leap to my death from its burning roof.

I don't voice this to the social worker.

I voice more specific worries. I'm worried I'm never going to feel better. I'm worried Anna is growing distant from me.

The social worker had a sister who died of cancer. Because she reveals that, I do not dismiss all her suggestions.

Suggestions I dismiss:

Set a timer, to limit wallowing in negative thoughts to ten minutes a day.

Consider purchasing a cute, fun purse, to hide that carry-along IV pump.

Read pamphlet about the importance of acceptance.

See hospital psychiatrist for a prescription for antidepressants.

Suggestions I try:

Set small achievable goals.

Initiate discussion with Anna regarding how she feels about my being sick.

I start one morning, when Anna and I are alone at the table, lingering over breakfast; her with a book, me with the newspaper.

"I'm sorry I missed spending time with you when I was in the hospital for so long. It made me feel angry. Did it make you angry?" I'm following the social worker's exact script. Anna looks up at me, one hand marking her place in her book.

"I saw you," she reminds me, "when I visited," and turns back to her book.

I try again, "Well, I'm hoping to spend a lot more time with you now."

She puts her book down this time and gives me a thumbs-up sign with both thumbs. And that's it. Our heart-to-heart took ten seconds. I'm not sure that's what the social worker had in mind.

To my surprise, it is Jack who initiates the next conversation, this time in the middle of dinner. I had said something in passing about a doctor's appointment.

"Does that mean me and Anna have a higher chance of getting it?" he asks calmly, as if it were purely theoretical and he is just asking out of curiosity. I stumble in my rush to tell him no, no, no. No one in my extended family has had this. It's random. He and Anna do not have any higher chance of getting it than anyone else. It is not hereditary.

But other things are. During a trip to England to visit Simon's family when they were six years old, Jack and Anna found the partially eaten body of a moorhen chick by the edge of a pond on Uncle Richard's property. They spent all afternoon burying it, and marking the site carefully with twigs and stones and feathers. Just before tea time, all the adults gathered in a semicircle around the grave, while Anna, hands folded in front of her, said a few words about what she thought the life of the little chick would have been like. I only remember the last line, "Little chick goodbye, who never got to fly." Maybe there is a funeral-planning gene.

I do better with setting small achievable goals: I play Anna's favorite card game, Slam, with her for the first time in a year; I watch recorded episodes of *The Daily Show*, with Jack and Simon; I start inviting friends over for morning visits.

In bed, however, I continue to fixate on what I've lost, rather than what I can achieve. I've always had trouble staying asleep, consumed as I was by the worries that nibble the night and gnaw at you in the darkness. But at least I never used to have trouble falling asleep. I used to drop instantly. Between saying the words, "good" and "night," to Simon, I was gone. Now I approach the shores of sleep warily, uneasily, like a refugee in a leaky boat. Even if I make it, will they let me stay? I'm weary. I'm exhausted. Still, sleep eludes me. It lies tantalizingly behind barbed-wire fences, and walls patrolled by guards. Even when I finally make it, it is not welcoming. Sleep is one more place where I no longer belong.

I've lost my will to live. More importantly, I've lost my narrative arc. I'm going nowhere. I'm constantly shuffling through the calendar in my mind. It's been seven months since I was diagnosed with leukemia. Five of those months I spent in hospitals. But now, all the treatments, the rounds of chemotherapy, the radiation, and the stem cell transplant, are finished. And finished successfully, as far as they can tell at this point anyway. You would think I would be celebrating. You would be wrong.

I read a book about cancer that includes the story of a man who was devastated when he was diagnosed with prostate cancer, and told he had only a 65 percent chance of surviving. I am sunk by the realization that I went through half a year of hell, just to *reach* a 65 percent chance of surviving; that my victory was to claw my way up to the worst moment in someone else's life.

What have I won? Life and death are not an all-or-nothing proposition like I had always thought. You can pay too high a price for life, and death is not always the worst possible outcome.

The messages from friends are congratulatory: You did it; hurray; way to go; you've been through hell, but now you're home! But I feel like I'm in a different kind of hell. A prison whose bars confining me are not the wheelchairs and beds and IV lines of the hospital wards, but fatigue, depression, pain, and most of all fear, fear, fear.

What are you afraid of?

I'm afraid I've been so absent from Jack and Anna that I'll never be able to make up for it and regain the important place I used to have in their lives; that the adjustment they have made because of my absence may be permanent.

I'm afraid that maybe being cured is not the same thing as being better. All this time, I thought it would be.

I'm afraid I won't drink enough water and will get so dehydrated I damage my kidneys. I will get an infection. The stem cells will attack all my organs, one by one. Or something else, I don't know what, will happen, and I'll have to go back to the hospital.

Anything else?

I'm afraid that because I'm so ungrateful, so horribly unappreciative of Simon, of my doctors, my donor, my mother, and everyone else, so unworthy of what so many people have done for me…the leukemia will come back.

I don't think it works like that.

What if it does, though? And what if…what if I never get back to my old self? What if, as exhausted and depressed as I am, this is how I will always be? What if I stay this way forever? What if I'm never fully alive again? What if I'm only this ghost, haunting the life I used to have? What if I would be better off dead?

Really? That's really what you think?

Fine, not *really*, really, just kind of really. I want my old life back. I won't accept this sad, damaged one. I won't, I won't, I won't.

Then don't.

"Wow," responds my friend Peter, when he reads a version of the above on CaringBridge. "Too bad your wallowing timer didn't go off before you wrote all *that*."

Most people, though, in their CaringBridge responses are warm and encouraging, chiming in about how wonderful I am, how brave. "Well, except maybe your mom," I muse to Simon, as I'm recounting to him the messages I've been getting. "She has more of a 'suck it up' tone."

"That's because she's being supportive of *me*," Simon points out.

CHAPTER TWENTY-THREE

MY HEAD is deep under the duvet, my IV pump is beeping again, and Simon is out grocery shopping. So when I hear someone call my name, I think I must be dreaming it. Then I hear it again, *Manjusha*.

I turn over heavily, one hand on my ileostomy bag, so I don't accidentally put my full weight on it. I push off my covers and prop myself up on one elbow so I can reach the IV stand. I click open the control panel and turn it off. I unhook one line to start flicking at the air bubbles. I had to learn how to do it myself, because Simon eventually got fed up and refused to come upstairs every time the alarm went off. The home care nurse, who comes every day to set up the bags, taught Simon how to unhook the lines when the bags are empty and how to flush the lines with heparin and wipe the caps, so the tubes going into my chest don't get blocked or infected. He also taught Simon what to do when the IV pump beeps. But Simon's had enough and thinks I'm capable of doing at least that much for myself.

Afternoons were never my favorite part of the day, but now I dread them. The residual optimism of the morning has crumbled, and the evening that marks the end of one more weary day is still an eternity away. The afternoon has no hope, and no momentum. Time stretches and sinks, and takes me with it. Simon keeps suggesting that the IV lines be hooked up while I'm downstairs, so I can sit in the family room, watch TV, read. But I refuse and hide. I reject distractions. I'm too busy being sad.

We're at a standoff.

"I'm going to stay in bed until I feel better," I say.

"If you stay in bed, you won't ever feel better" is Simon's response, more stern than sympathetic.

He indulged me when I was in physical pain, but no longer. You have to eat, you have to sit up, you have to walk, you have to participate. He's urging me to try. I'm wishing for a pill that will put me to sleep until all this is over. Neither of us is getting what we want. But by leaving me alone in the afternoon, something he has never done before, he's forcing me to deal with the IV pump myself, for the first time.

Intent on flicking the line, and watching the air bubbles slowly rise back up to the bag, I forget about the voice, until it calls out again, more insistently: *Manjusha*. I glance over at my crowded night table. There's my clock radio. It's not on. There's my iPod, the earbuds dangling precariously off the edge. Some crumpled-up Kleenex. A few individual squares of alcohol wipes. A stack of books. A small bowl of cashews, today's afternoon snack.

Simon insists I eat something every few hours, since I can't manage anything much at meals. I've thrown most of the cashews away, carefully wrapping them in toilet paper first, so no one sees them in the bathroom trash can. I left a few though, as I always do, for the sake of believability. Simon will be suspicious if the bowl is completely empty.

There's my small sculpture of Ganesh, the god of wisdom; the intricately carved lines a dusty white against the gray stone. It's my most treasured possession. I love the calm expression on his face, the comfortable weight of the stone in my palm, cool and smooth to the touch. Wait a minute, I blink, he lives on my desk at work, not at home. But I look again, and there he is, reclining at his ease as usual, one ankle hooked over the other, an open book resting on his plump belly. His elephant head is turned away from me.

His mother, the goddess Parvati, created him to guard her chamber while she bathed. When her husband, Lord Shiva, tried to enter, Ganesh confronted him and was beheaded for his efforts. But when Lord Shiva saw how much this distressed Parvati, he gave Ganesh an elephant head as a replacement, along with powers that made Ganesh the most appealed to of all the gods, because he can remove obstacles, relieve suffering, and bestow happiness.

I realize he's the one who called my name.

He's never spoken to me before.

Should I answer back? Should I tell him what I want? I want to be healthy, of course. Wait, I don't just want to be restored to health. I want never to have been sick. And I want never to be sick in the future. But I don't want to live forever. I want to live, let's see, ninety healthy years (one hundred, though a more satisfyingly round number, seems greedy and, frankly, too long) and then I want to die painlessly, in my sleep, with no advance warning. And I want all my family and all my friends to be healthy and happy. Oh, but I do want the memory of this (can I have the memory without the experience? Why not, right?), so I remember to be kind when people around me are mean or angry, sad or scared. And also so I don't get annoyed if I have to wait too long in line for something.

Okay.

Okay, as in it's okay to want this, or okay, as in okay you're going to grant this?

Just okay.

Oh I know, you're going to say yes, but first bring me a handful of salt from a house, blah blah blah.

Yes never has a but. And that wasn't me.

Wasn't me who?

Wasn't me who said yes, but first bring me a handful of salt.

Fine, magical mustard seed then, whatever. You're going to say first bring me a mustard seed from a household that has never known sorrow.

Magical mustard seed? That's the Chinese version. Magical mustard seed indeed. Doesn't exist. But every household has salt. Besides, they're both a trick. I don't trick people.

I don't know. What about when you won that bet with your brother? About who could travel around the world the fastest? Wasn't that a trick?

No. Your parents are your world, so when you circle them in prayer, you've gone around your world. It's a common custom; a gesture of respect; a metaphor. Metaphors are not tricks. I'm the other salt story.

There's another salt story?

There are a million salt stories. Gandhi defeated the British Empire with a handful of—

I know, I know. I saw the movie.

—salt. This is the one about the guru and the complaining disciple who walk into a bar. Stop me if you've heard it already. No? Well, the disciple is in a lot of pain and wants the guru to help him. The guru, that's me by the way, gives him a handful of salt, tells him to mix it in a glass of water and drink it, and then asks him how it tastes. The disciple says, Awful. The guru then gives him another handful of salt, tells him to throw it into the lake and take a glass of lake water and drink it, and then asks him how that tastes. The disciple says, Sweet.

I get it.

See, you can't change the pain, but you can change the receptacle.

I said, I get it.

You can dilute the suffering. You can be the lake.

Okay, okay, but what about the elephant? Who lost his head for you? What about his suffering?

Hmm. Stories differ.

How surprising.

Either he sacrificed himself willingly to help my father, or my father had to slay him in battle and gain his head as the prize. Either way.

Either way what?

Either way. You win, and there's some price. You lose, and there's some gain. In exchange for one elephant's suffering, some say that all elephants now get to enter the Kingdom of the Gods.

But I don't believe in gods. I believe in stories.

Either way.
This again?
If there are no stories, there are no gods.

CHAPTER TWENTY-FOUR

MY ILEOSTOMY BAG is leaking. I'm sitting at the dining room table, trying to eat some cereal, when I feel its contents oozing out where the seal has pulled away from my skin. I clutch it to my stomach and walk gingerly to the kitchen to rifle through the basket that contains my medications, pamphlets, phone numbers. I call my home care nurse, Yuri, on his cell. He's my favorite nurse, and I can count on him, day or night. I'm breathless and panicky when I reach him. He's not due to come by for a few hours, but he says he'll try to come earlier.

I go upstairs, take a hand towel to cover the bag, and lie flat on my bed to wait for him. I wriggle the sheets down, so I don't make a mess. If life hands you lemons, make lemonade. But what if life hands you a bag of your own shit? Can you make something out of that?

I feel like I'm holding my breath until he arrives. I'm so

grateful when I hear his voice greeting Simon at the front door. Soon, I hear his heavy steps on the stairs, and he comes in. He's put those blue sanitary socks over his shoes, and he goes to the bathroom to wash his hands before approaching me, his cheeks ruddy from the cold, above his graying beard.

"Let's see," he says, removing the towel that covers my bag. "Yes, it has lifted off." He tsks as he peels the rest of it away and puts it in a garbage bag. "But skin good, not red." He briskly cleans the stoma, flaps to dry it, and sticks on another flange and bag.

"Why is it doing that?" I ask plaintively. "You just changed it yesterday. I thought it was supposed to last a week." Although I have to empty the bag every couple of hours, I was told in the hospital that the bag itself only had to be changed every six to ten days. He shrugs.

"May be the medication you are on. Is paste you can get. If I have, I will bring next time. Or you can order, stoma paste, helps with seal." He goes to the office and wheels the IV stand into the bedroom and starts attaching the bags.

Yuri is originally from Siberia. I was surprised when he first told me that. I had pictured Siberia as a frozen wasteland (perhaps how many people picture Canada). I knew it only as a place that Russia sent prisoners and political dissidents. I didn't know that regular people lived there. He was an oral surgeon and his wife was a gynecologist.

"We make only twenty-four dollars each month," he told me. "I make more when we first move to Canada and I work at gas station. My daughter, she was six years old when we leave. In Siberia we can afford for her only one apple, maybe, in a week. My friends move to Israel, say you come too. But I like cold, not hot, so we come to Canada."

He's the only immigrant I know who doesn't complain about the winter. He and his wife both work as home care nurses, but he is writing his exams to qualify as a dentist. Once he qualifies, his wife will then write her exams. His daughter just started first-year science at the University of Toronto, and he now also has a son who is six years old.

"I have a question." He hooks the first bag to the stand. "Because always I see books everywhere here. I want to ask, can you recommend for my daughter. I want books for her, about love, about how to live."

"How to live?" I'm not sure what he means.

"Yes, you know, to teach the best about love, life, what a young woman should know."

"Does she like to read?" I ask.

"Oh yes, she reads a lot, mostly for school."

"*The Book Thief?*" For some reason it's the first one that comes to mind.

"Mmm." He hesitates. "She has read this one, I think. She liked it very much."

My fantasy has come true, someone is asking me for a book prescription. But Yuri's request is both too difficult and too easy. Aren't all books about life and love? I think I know what he means, though, something beautiful, something inspiring.

"*Captain Corelli's Mandolin,*" I start again, "by Louis de Bernières. *History of Love* by Nicole Krauss. Umm…" Why is this so hard? "And, and, *Lives of Girls and Women* by Alice Munro."

The last is more moving than inspiring, but shouldn't I have something real as well, and shouldn't I have something Canadian? I don't know why that's important to me. Am I selecting a politically correct syllabus for a first-year English course or am I trying to give some helpful recommendations to my home care nurse? He's entering the names on his phone as I give them. I spell Louis de Bernières for him.

When he leaves, I start having second thoughts. I can't believe I forgot *Middlemarch*, one of my favorite books of all time. And I'm feeling unsure about *Captain Corelli*, though I was obsessed with that book for years. I even edited down a passage from it about love and recited it at several friends' weddings, and a friend read it at my own; about how love is when the two of you have roots that grow toward each other underground, and when all the pretty blossoms have fallen from your branches, you find that you are one tree, and not two. I used to think that was so perfect.

I don't think that anymore.

Love is not a tree, because trees die. Love is a rock. And not stone that crumbles into dust. It's the Canadian Shield itself, granite as old as the Earth, solid and unwavering beneath my weak and unsteady feet.

I detest not only my ileostomy bag, but all my pills as well, cyclosporine most of all. Gray, greasy, and vile smelling, the smooth oval pills come in blister-packed perforated strips. I have to take five in the morning and five at bedtime. They make me feel queasy and troubled.

"I can't do it." I gag after taking one and pace around the bedroom a few times to try to get rid of the feeling that I'm going to throw it back up again. I still have four more to go.

"I don't want to take them anymore." I am now leaning on the dresser looking in the mirror at the reflection of Simon, behind me, reading in bed.

"Then don't," he says, not even looking up from his book.

I'm taken aback. "What do you mean 'don't'?"

"I mean don't. You can stop taking them."

"No, I can't," I sputter. "I have to take them to get better."

"Then you want to take them."

I frown, but before I can object, he continues, "Manjusha, that's how you have to think of it."

The minute she reads my CaringBridge post about my struggles with cyclosporine, Kathie calls me.

"That's my fungus!" she says.

"What do you mean, that's your fungus?"

"It's the one I identified, that got all the publicity."

"When you went on *Good Morning America?*" I'm excited because I think I remember it all now.

"Well, I didn't go. It went by itself, without me."

"But it's yours, you discovered it!"

"I didn't discover it." She tries to explain as simply as she can.

At the time Kathie made her finding, cyclosporine was already being used to suppress the immune systems of transplant patients. Pharmaceutical companies had developed the drug from a chemical they found in a fungus they actually knew very little about. Kathie describes the fungus to me as looking like "a bit of white fluff" on the forest floor. That fluffy fungus produces a chemical that helps it invade insects, so it can kill and feed off them.

One day, while Kathie's class was on a woodland foray, a student brought her a little fungus that hadn't been seen in the Ithaca area before. It was killing a beetle. Kathie took it to her lab and grew it in a petri dish. She found that this beetle-killing fungus, when it grew in her lab, turned into the white fluffy cyclosporine-making fungus.

Nobody had connected the two before. They were thought to be two completely different fungi. Apparently, you need to know what a fungi's flowering state is, to know what it's related to, and where it belongs on the Tree of Life, whose branches cover all living things: animals, plants, and fungi. As a result of this finding, money was raised to set aside land as a biodiversity preserve, and a drug company funded a bio-prospecting project to look for other fungi that could have medicinal properties. And, what had stuck in my mind, the fungus itself made an appearance on the breakfast talk show *Good Morning America*.

"It's like," she searches for a way to help me grasp it, "it's like, it's as if we knew there were butterflies, and we knew there were caterpillars, but we never knew they were connected. And now we know." I want to ask her which the cyclosporine is, the butterfly or the caterpillar, but I decide the analogy probably doesn't stretch that far. Anyway, it's as much information as I need. My unpleasant little pills suddenly seem full of fluttering personality.

Even when I'm finally weaned off them, after months of the dosages decreasing, increasing, and decreasing again, I still feel a jolt of interest whenever I'm in the waiting room of the transplant clinic and I see someone take out the telltale foil strip of pills. I'm so tempted to sidle over and ask confidingly, "Do you want to hear something completely fascinating…?"

CHAPTER TWENTY-FIVE

I ENTER the Queen's Landing Hotel reception area at Niagara-on-the-Lake for a work-related conference. It's my first large event in more than a year. Heads swivel, eyes flicker toward me, my head wrapped in a bright silk scarf, my face round and puffy from the steroids. I am pitied, I am admired. I am doomed, I am destined. I am battered, I am beautiful. I am cursed, I am blessed. I hum with possibility, good and bad. I am assigned virtues, I am forgiven sins. I am not half anything, my glass is drained, it is full to overflowing. I can see people trying to work out if I am the luckiest or the unluckiest person they know.

I scare you, I reassure you. When you fill me in on what's been happening with you, you preface every story of broken bones and cancer scares with a humble "I know it's nothing compared with what you've been through." I like to win, but this is a contest I wish I never had to enter. You count your lucky stars, there but for the grace of whatever…. You cling to your children a little tighter. You wonder if the end of life as you know it is too high a price to pay for the chance to start a new one. I am ancient, I am reborn. I am considered brave because I am breathing. I am a rock star.

I actually receive applause just for being alive. Whenever someone approaches me with arms warmly extended, my colleague Ann throws her arm in front of me like a parent does to a child when the car brakes suddenly. No hugs. She has spent the previous half hour in my hotel room wiping down all the surfaces with the hand sanitizer she packed especially for this purpose: tap handles, toilet flush, door knobs, telephone, TV remote.

She collects me for breakfast and tells me she realized suddenly in the middle of the night that breakfast would be a buffet. A buffet! Touching a serving spoon would be like shaking hands with all 200 people in attendance at the conference. All previous precautions would have been for nothing. She serves me after I point out which pieces of bacon I want, which slices of French toast. I'm a preemie in an incubator, a woman in a niqab, a tiger in a cage. You can't touch me.

It took a while to obtain medical permission to attend that conference. I don't mean a while for me to get strong enough to withstand the risk of infection, I mean a while until I found a doctor who said it was okay. My mantra of "small, achievable goals" gradually becomes more ambitious and crafty, despite frequent setbacks. When I moan at one appointment about my lack of progress, with the cyclosporine going tantalizingly down almost to zero and then right back up to ten pills a day, that day's doctor tells me, "You're a yo-yo on an up-going escalator," and I cling to that image.

I sign up for, and then cancel, my registration at an exercise program for cancer patients several times, until my doctors say I'm stable enough to go. Permission to swim in fresh water, the cool clear rivers and lakes I've been dreaming about being in ever since I got sick, takes another whole year, though not for lack of repeated requests. The first time I ask if I can return to work, the answer is a sarcastic, but kind "Sure, and then you'll work for five minutes and be off sick for six months," which I take as a no. Permission to go to a nail salon never comes, and I don't bother pursuing it. I'm prepared to risk getting sick for work or for swimming, but not for a pedicure.

The day I start my exercise class at Wellspring, on the grounds of Sunnybrook Hospital, I discreetly eye the other participants to determine where I am in relation to them. I'm disappointed to find I don't come off well in my comparisons. Half seem on the older, frailer side and half on the younger, fitter side. I feel like I don't fit in either category, because I'm younger than the oldsters, but frailer than the youngsters. I'm the only one wearing a cancer cap. I envy the thick hair of the women I chat with before the class begins. You know it's bad when you're jealous of women who have breast cancer.

At my intake assessment, Nicole notes down my resting blood pressure, oxygen level, heart rate, and weight. She gets me to clench a small metal vise to check my grip strength and asks me to balance for one minute, on one leg at a time.

I can't do it. She comes up with a program for me, one that alternates between cardio and strengthening exercises. She warns me not to overdo it. "You have to listen to your body," she says. I want to tell her that my body and I are no longer on speaking terms, ever since it tried to kill me all those months ago, but I don't.

The cardio is gentle—hallway walk, stationary bike, treadmill, only for three minutes at a time. The room is bright and new, lined on one side with windows, with trees blocking the view of the hospital across the various parking areas. The instructors glow with health and friendliness. There is music playing in the background when I start gently bouncing on a tiny trampoline, "I'm on my way, from misery to happiness today…" My heart bounds. I'm sure it's a sign. Eventually, I realize it's not a sign, but a CD, one they play at every single class. But still, I never get sick of that particular chorus.

I enthusiastically check out program after program at Wellspring. First, a drop-in yoga class, where I blame my complete lack of flexibility (I can't even sit cross-legged) on the cancer and ileostomy, when really I suspect I was never very bendy even before. Then a dance yoga session where Simon is appalled to learn that we sing a song (with actions!) about how when you send joy, joy, joy, out into the world, world, world, it all comes back to you, you, you (appalled because 1. He was actually considering going with me and, 2. I love the song and insist on singing it for days after). I even check out a couple of dry-sounding sessions about long-term disability benefits.

There are also cooking classes I consider attending, but never get around to. "Healthy snacks" seem oxymoronic, like "jumbo shrimp," but way less delicious. One time, walking past the class kitchen, I hear an excited, "I can't believe this drink has lentils in it!" Me neither, I silently respond as I speed thankfully by. I still eat bacon, because otherwise the cancer wins. But I do decide it's time to stop the Diet Coke, as I'm concerned about the aspartame Jack is always warning me about. Simon is incredulous when he sees the shopping list I leave on the counter for him, a few weeks after I start at Wellspring.

"That's your idea of making a healthy change?" he asks. "Switching from Diet Coke to regular Coke?"

"I only drink half the can," I say defensively.

"Great, you can use the other half to clean the toilet."

"Very funny," I scoff. "Like I ever clean anything."

I have to take an extended break from the program for my ileostomy reversal and recovery. The same amazing surgeon who saved me with the emergency ileostomy does the reversal. She calls me a "tough cookie" for surviving the first surgery. I tell her what I am most afraid of.

"Homer says I should wait, in case I get cancer again, and have to do the operation all over."

She shrugs. "Everybody's going to get cancer."

The surgery goes perfectly, but still I cannot resume the exercise class until months later. During these months, I have to go for daily appointments so a nurse can change my surgical dressings, check that the openings where the intestine ends poked out have healed, and remove the staples from the six-inch incision. The intervening time is long enough that Nicole's partner has not only given birth to their baby boy, but they've even taken said baby on a trip to Australia. I give her a signed copy of my children's book as a baby gift. She's delighted, and even more delighted with the progress I've made. At my reassessment, I weigh more, grip harder, balance on each foot with ease, and stride forcefully up and down the hallway.

"Okay, you've got ten weeks left, let's set some goals." We're in the ante room sitting across from each other on comfy chairs.

"I want to be as strong as it is humanly possible to be," I say immediately.

She laughs, pauses, and then writes down, "Increase heart rate to over 150 during cardio intervals."

"Next goal?" she asks.

"I want never to get sick again," I answer.

"Improve posture," she writes down.

There's a whole new group of people in my second go-round at Wellspring, and this time I'm in the vigorous half. I've even stopped wearing my cancer scarf; while my hair is not great, being self-conscious about the thinness is still better than wearing the cap or the itchy wig I briefly tried. Nicole keeps adding things to my routine, five minutes on the elliptical machine, a dozen pulls on the wall-mounted stretchy thing.

"I have a great idea for you," she tells me one morning, instead of saying hello. I'm expecting something new involving the exercise ball, but it's an idea for a children's book.

"You should write one where the kid just happens to have two moms, you know, but it's not the point of the story. You know what I mean?"

"Totally," I say fervently. "I hate when the only time you

see a kid in a wheelchair, say, is when the whole book is about that. That's why, you know, in my story, Meena's Indian but it's not about that, it's about how she hates books. She just happens to be Indian."

"That's what I'm talking about!" Nicole is pleased I understand what she means. I'm pleased we're not talking about exercising.

CHAPTER TWENTY-SIX

WHAT I FIRST want to write, though, is a better metaphor for my cancer. I'm a sucker for a good metaphor. One afternoon when Simon and I were sitting in the family room with my parents, a coyote actually walked up the ravine, right to our back door. He was more imposing, and more golden, than I had thought a coyote would be. He sniffed around the garden and driveway for a few minutes and then disappeared back into the ravine. My friend Casey told me it was a sign and wrote on CaringBridge, "My great-grandmother Kathleen used to say, if a golden coyote walks up to your door, it's time to get a bigger purse for all the good fortune that's coming your way. Be prepared." When I mention to him, months later, how much I liked that image, he just looks at me. "I made that up," he says.

When we were looking into special science and math high school programs, Jack and I attended several open houses.

I liked the one for the TOPS program at Marc Garneau Collegiate Institute the best, simply because of a metaphor.

One of the science teachers spoke passionately about how, unlike the Jack of Jack and the Beanstock fame (who killed the giant), they wanted to help free our children's inner giants, unleashing their full potential, letting their true selves burst forth and conquer the world. I just ate that up. One parent I spoke to was dismissive about how the school didn't provide stats on how many of their students got into Harvard compared to students at other high schools. But I didn't care. I don't want statistics. I want coyotes bringing good luck, and children becoming giants.

Metaphors are transformative, changing something into something else, something better. For me, the best way to understand something is to think of it in terms of something else. But cancer eludes me. It is cells in my body. It is stars in the sky. It's a crab. It's a killer. You can have it. You can be it. It has metaphors. It *is* a metaphor. Homer, you told me cells don't have motivations, but I give you Exhibit A, the *Canadian Oxford Dictionary*. How many other diseases have "evil" in their definition?

> **cancer *n*. 1 a** any malignant growth or tumour from an abnormal and uncontrolled division of body cells. **b** a disease characterized by this. **2** an evil influence or corruption spreading uncontrollably. **3 (Cancer)** a constellation between Gemini and Leo, tradition- ally regarded as contained in the figure of a crab. **4 (Cancer) a** the fourth sign of the zodiac. **b** a person born when the sun is in this sign, usu. between 21 June and 22 July.

The metaphor for cancer as a war comes in for a lot of flak (but clearly it's an irresistible one, as I can't even criticize it without using it). The criticism is mainly that battles have winners and losers, and it's not fair to say someone lost their battle with cancer, because it implies that they were deficient in some way…that they were to blame. If they had been stronger, tougher, more positive, they would have been a winner and not a loser. Obviously this is not fair. It is not your fault if you die of cancer.

If you dare put I "battled" cancer in my obituary, one letter-to-the-editor writer expounds, I will come back to haunt you.

I read attempts to come up with other metaphors. A psychiatrist suggests it is a conversation, an attempt to communicate, to mediate, with cancer cells, to calm them and slow them down. A science writer suggests it is a dance where no one's winning or losing, we're in this together. But I'm not fighting, or talking, or dancing (despite my first idea that my chromosomes were changing places like square dance partners). I'm enduring.

Homer's description of it as a marathon is the one I find most apt. When he first said it, I didn't like it because I was feeling upbeat and didn't want to think about how far I still had to go. But later, he uses it more encouragingly.

"It's a marathon, but you'll get through it," he says.

"A marathon in hell," I grumble. Because normally you're not forced to run a marathon, you choose to run it. But there is a choice here as well, albeit not a very palatable one. You could not engage, you could sit it out, but then you'd never make it to the finish line. You may not make it if you try either, but you definitely won't if you don't try. And unlike a war, you're not fighting, you're enduring. You're putting your head down and concentrating on dragging one foot forward at a time.

After the stem cell transplant, I figured I was almost at the finish line, but instead of feeling good, I was feeling worse than ever. "The closer you get to the end, the worse you feel," Homer explained consolingly. "That's when it's the hardest, that's when you want to die." And it is. Even though you can see the end, instead of inspiring you, it seems to taunt you. *Ha ha, still not there, still feel like crap. You could come this far and still not make it.* I was filled with optimism at the beginning but it was really ignorance. I was hopeful only because I had no idea how hopeless it would feel.

The poets were wrong, or at least partly wrong. It *is* Time you always hear at your back, but Time is not gliding along on a winged chariot, which I picture as all golden and borne along by the wind. Time is clutching a walker, shuffle-scraping behind you along an endless hospital corridor, reminding you that worse than the fear of death is the fear of the stretched-out dying that comes before, the smell of the stacked trays of leftover hospital meals in the hallway, the nausea, the pain, the weariness, the ugliness.

I go back to the idea of a battle, or more than a battle, an all-out unconventional war, where no option is too extreme.

ACT ONE

The curtain rises on a classic Hollywood-esque Situation Room. A dozen people sit around a long table, crowded with computers. Screens line the walls.

CHIEF OF DEFENSE: Commander, we have a situation.

SECURITY ANALYST #1: Good thing we're in the Situation Room then, isn't it?

SECURITY ANALYST #2: *(Snorts.)*

CHIEF OF DEFENSE *(continuing, as if no one has spoken)*: Terrorist cells have been identified.

(A murmur passes around the table.)

COMMANDER: How many?

CHIEF OF DEFENSE *(pauses, and murmuring trails off)*: Thousands. No, more like millions.

COMMANDER: Millions? Millions?? How could that many get past us? Why wasn't I notified earlier?

CHIEF OF DEFENSE: We just found out. It—

COMMANDER: Just found out? How could—

CHIEF OF DEFENSE: Commander, please, one moment. You'll see. We just found out because they didn't get *past* us. They *are* us. Troops gone rogue, homegrown terrorism, whatever the hell you want to call it.

COMMANDER *(without hesitating)*: You know the drill. Fire away.

(Everyone exits quickly. Cut to the next scene, in the same Situation Room, but it is dark. Only the computer screens glow. The COMMANDER and CHIEF OF DEFENSE are the only ones in the room.)

COMMANDER: Well?

CHIEF OF DEFENSE *(wearily)*: Firepower was great. Damage was greater. And...

COMMANDER: And?

CHIEF OF DEFENSE: It was not successful.

COMMANDER: So, our nuclear option is the only one remaining?

CHIEF OF DEFENSE: Unfortunately, yes. But—

COMMANDER: But what?

CHIEF OF DEFENSE: You are sure troops from outside

will come in? To rebuild? After? Will they? Otherwise, it's pointless. Isn't it?

COMMANDER *(shrugging)*: It might be pointless if we act. But it's definitely pointless if we don't. They've confirmed. That's all I can say. It's not like we'll be around to follow up.

CHIEF OF DEFENSE: Some of our troops could show them.

COMMANDER: You know none of our troops will sur—

"I don't think this 'cancer cells as terrorists' thing works," Simon objects. "Plus, it's full of clichés."

"What do you mean?" I ask. "I thought it was perfect. Cancer cells are powerful, they're destructive. They're immune to reason, even to save themselves. Get it? And the clichés are there on purpose, because I'm trying to mimic—"

"Wait a minute," Simon protests, "I never criticized it." He's objecting to his first objection, which, I have to admit, I did sort of make up.

"Are you sure?" I ask, not willing to concede that I made it up. "When I told you about it that time we were walking? Didn't you say it was a stretch?"

"I did not." He is adamant.

"But I can't just float a whole huge metaphor like that without an accompanying critique!"

"Well, critique it yourself." He is refusing to play along,

demonstrating what I think is a rather literal adherence to the notion that a memoir is completely true.

"But the critique would be so much better if it was in the form of a dialogue," I argue. "I can't have a conversation with myself."

"Most of your conversations are with yourself," he points out, accurately enough.

I run the metaphor by Homer since he was a colonel in the Canadian Forces Health Services. He is skeptical.

"No one would ever, ever authorize a nuclear attack on their own troops," he informs me.

"Even if it was absolutely the only way to defeat the enemy forces?"

"No way. They would never purposely bomb everyone and risk destroying the whole country so new troops could come in and rebuild."

("Or at least they would never *say* that's what they were doing" is Simon's contribution, on the record).

"But that's what they did to me, isn't it? With the chemo and radiation and transplant? Wasn't that the nuclear option? Kill every single one of my white blood cells, good and bad, even though there was a pretty high chance it could kill me? And then send in someone else's blood cells to rebuild from scratch?"

Homer pauses, and then admits that this is, indeed, what they did to me.

My pride in my metaphor is short-lived. I am sobered by the realization that the war against cancer is more vicious than a classic war would be. In this war, there are no Geneva conventions; nuclear strikes against your own citizens are the only options. And, after everything, I don't even get to claim the victory myself. Because I wasn't the one fighting the battle. I was only the battleground, the miles of territory won and lost, and won again. But the full debrief, the complete accounting, is still to come at some unknown time in the future. Until then, I will know neither the extent of the victory nor its price.

CHAPTER TWENTY-SEVEN

THE PHONE RINGS, jolting me out of the fast asleepness of my afternoon nap. The duvet is as heavy and warm over my head as the afternoon is chilly and gray. The phone is on Simon's side of the bed, because that's where the jack is, not because Simon ever wants to use it, and the message is already half over before I can even contemplate stretching out to reach it.

"...Dr. G.'s office, please call back at..." I'll call back later I think, about to sink back into my nap, and then something niggles at me and I am suddenly wide awake. Why is Dr. G.'s office calling me? It could only be one reason. He had sent me for a mammogram and breast ultrasound this week, part of the ongoing monitoring for secondary cancers because of all the radiation I had. He must have the test results. And it's a quick leap from that to, if he's calling, the results must be bad. They never call with good news. In fact, I was expecting to have to call in the next week or so, just to follow up, so sure was I that they would not call me. I grab the phone to call back, get voice mail, and leave a message; but my peaceful afternoon is shot. I call back compulsively every half hour for the rest of the afternoon, but continue to get only voice mail. I don't leave any more messages.

"You don't know that it's bad news," says Simon.

"What else could it be?" I wail. I have breast cancer. Tears spring to my eyes. This is so unfair. Really. I can't have leukemia *and* breast cancer. Can I? It's getting ridiculous. Like Oscar Wilde saying losing one parent is a misfortune, losing both looks like carelessness; getting cancer is a tragedy, to keep getting it is a farce. One of those times where you start losing the sympathy you initially inspired, and start feeling like this is really reflecting badly on you. What lengths am I prepared to go to for attention, to keep the spotlight trained upon me, to keep the casseroles and gifts coming that have dried up of late? At some point it's no longer going to be sad, but unseemly.

Simon is sanguine. "You have bigger things to worry about," he reminds me. This does not help.

I have an appointment with my family doctor the next day for five vaccinations. When you have a stem cell transplant it's like you are reborn, so you have to have all the immunizations an infant would get in the first two years of life. I had been dreading it, but it now feels like a fun morning in comparison to what I fear lies ahead. I can't do more chemo. I won't, I won't, I won't. I ask my doctor if she has the ultrasound results, suddenly thinking maybe, just maybe, the clinic faxed them to her. She checks, but they weren't sent to her since she wasn't the doctor who requisitioned the tests.

I have to wait an endless two weeks to get an appointment to go over the test results. Then hours more to see the specialist, because he's late arriving at his clinic, due to an emergency at the hospital he attends. When I finally see the test results, I have to read the short paragraph several times before I understand that all it means is I have to repeat the test in six more months. The doctor does a quick manual check. "I think you just have lumpy breasts," he concludes reassuringly, albeit unflatteringly. Six months it is, and in six months it's fine.

I have a similar scare with a pap smear that sends me back to Sunnybrook for further testing that reveals "pre-cancerous" cervical cells. They are scraped out by laser in a very painful procedure, the start of which leaves me so tense and tearful they suggest doing it under general anesthetic. But that scares me more, so I say to go ahead and do it with local freezing. It turns out the set-up was the worst part, and the procedure itself is not that bad. I'm offered the chance to watch it on the screen. I decline. "Breathe deeply, stop twitching your toes," the doctor says, "because it makes your whole body move and you need to be still for the surgery." I stop.

I have to watch the nervous fidgeting. A while ago, a doctor, noticing my jiggling leg, got me a percussive MRI in the middle of the night to make sure I didn't have a brain tumor. I didn't. But it was lots of fun waiting to find out if I did.

Then I have a few instances when I have trouble catching my breath, and Simon marches me to emerg over my protests. I'm told I need another bronchoscopy. I won't do it. I won't do it. I have to do it.

It ends up being okay. I get a drug called "twilight" this time around and don't feel a thing. "It's what Michael Jackson used!" the nurse tells me cheerfully, even though that didn't work out so well for him. It turns out I don't have a fungal infection.

"Every time I get a cough now, I worry I'm dying," I complain to Simon.

"Get used to it" is all he says. "I've been doing that for thirty years."

I'm troubled that he still feels that way when his cancer was thirty years ago, but I'm reassured that he is here having this conversation *thirty years* later.

"I'm not a hypochondriac," I tell Kate on the phone, when she calls to check in on how I'm doing. "But now, after every test, I assume I'm going to die."

"It's post-traumatic stress disorder," she suggests.

"No, no, that's for veterans who've seen friends blown up beside them."

"No," she keeps going, "you're in a heightened state of anxiety. Something small happens, like having to repeat a test, and you assume the worst, because that's what it triggers. Your life was at risk. Like when a firecracker makes a soldier assume it's a bomb."

Battle metaphors, yet again. I need something better.

I decide to ask my mother if there's some Hindu myth that could work as a metaphor for cancer. My brother and I used to devour those luridly illustrated Amar Chitra Katha comic books as kids. There were so many heroes and heroines who cheated death, there must be something there.

She's not quite sure what I'm looking for.

"Some story where someone defeats death in some way," I explain vaguely. I decide I want a positive metaphor this time.

My brother and I have been rolling our eyes our whole childhood at her dinnertime dissertations about how Hinduism is misunderstood in the West; how people think it's about these hundreds of strange gods and goddesses, when really the stories represent great philosophical truths, blah blah blah. I can't believe that now that I actually want to listen to all that, she can't think of anything. She can't believe it either. She starts getting stressed, and frowning, as she struggles to come up with something.

"How about Krishna?" I ask impatiently. "Wasn't he going to get killed and then he escaped? Or something?"

"Yes!" Her eyes light up and she sits up straighter on the sofa she had slumped into as she was thinking. "Okay, so Kansa—"

"Who?"

"Kansa, the bad king, hears a prophecy that his sister's eighth son will defeat him. So he locks up his sister and sister's husband. They have no children yet, and he kills each child she has and—"

"Wait," I interrupt. "He kills seven babies?"

"Yes, and Krishna is eighth and he gets out. He gets smuggled out, and—"

"How is seven dead babies a story about defeating death?"

"No, no, point is *Krishna's* alive. When he's born, they switch him with a baby, a, a baby just born to some woodcutter and his wife, a baby girl, and they take the baby girl back to the jail. And then she, she ascends to heaven, triumphant, and says Ha! You didn't succeed, Krishna is still alive."

"Ascends to heaven? How is that triumphant? Doesn't that mean she died?"

"Umm yes, but see, Krishna won, that's the victory!" My mother pumps both fists in the air, presumably to illustrate what a great victory it was, but her arms drop down to her sides again when she sees my skeptical face.

"When we heard the story," she says, "we just thought, Yay! Krishna won. That's the point of it, that he tricked Kansa. But if I look at it your way, I see uh..." Her voice trails off.

"We were just really happy Krishna won," she repeats more strongly.

I am not convinced. That's not the kind of defeating death story I had in mind. Plus, Simon's busy poking more holes in it. "Why would Kansa lock his sister and her husband up together?" he asks me. I try again.

"Isn't there one about a wife? A wife whose husband dies, but then she follows him, and wins him back, or something?"

My mother nods eagerly. "Savitri and Satyavan!"

"Satya what?" I ask. I was hoping for a catchier name, so the story would be easier to follow.

"*Satya*van," she repeats, emphasizing the first syllable, and then tells me what she remembers of the story. I think it might work. I decide to save Satyavan for my epilogue.

CHAPTER TWENTY-EIGHT

I EVENTUALLY PROGRESS from the Princess Margaret dental clinic back to my own dentist. He's pleased to see me after all this time, and all I have been through. His usual practice is to check in briefly after the hygienist finishes her cleaning, but this time he stays longer, to hear how I'm doing. He shakes his head. "We are all tested in this life," he says solemnly, in response to my update.

If this is a test, I decide I don't think much of it. When I had imagined being tested for bravery all those years ago, I had meant in a shining flame of self-sacrifice and glory. I had not pictured a seemingly endless marathon of pointless suffering. That was the real disappointment. That I was enduring all of this without a reason, without benefiting anyone. What is the point of a test like that?

Then I realize I'm not *being* tested, I *am* the test. I'm not the person stepping in front of the speeding car, or bullet, I'm the person being saved. There are many heroes in this story, but none of them are me.

There are various lessons that could come out of grappling with a life-threatening illness: be more kind; be more patient; spend more time with your family and less time at work. Some of the lessons work against each other. Should you seize the day, or should you stop and smell the roses? You cannot do both. Life is short. Make every second count, but how? By doing more or by doing less?

All I want is to have my exact same life back, and to be exactly the person I was. Of course I would like to be a better person, but not with this price tag. I don't want a sneak preview of the hell that is in store for me. I want to forget I ever had the glimpse that I did. I don't want to prove that now I can wait patiently for that dim sum cart to arrive. I'm writing a book not to exorcise demons, but to be able to say "Oh yes, that time I wrote that book," not "Oh that time that I had cancer." Isn't it enough that a random bad thing happened? Does it also have to redefine who I am?

"What's the moral here?" Marge Simpson asks. I'm with Homer when he answers, "It's just a bunch of stuff that happened."

I'm not braver, or more patient, or more resigned to fate. I thought I would be. A radio producer, while prepping me for an interview about stem cell transplants, asks if this experience has changed me as a person. She doesn't say "for the better," but I know that is implied. Suddenly I'm angry. No, I say slowly and evenly, trying not to sound upset. I'm not a better person now because of my brush with death. In fact, I want to say that it seems really, really unfair to me that not only do I have to face the pain and trauma and terror of cancer, but I *also* have to work at being a better person as a result. It's taking all I have just to try to get back to the person that I was, to do the things I always loved to do. If I can do that, I will be so grateful. Do I really have to do more than that? Isn't that hard enough to grasp?

"Let's do bird puns," Jack begs. We've just gotten out of the car at a conservation area east of Toronto. Anna scuttles out of earshot with Simon; they're not fans of puns.

"Okay," I say. "I went first last time, now it's your tern."

"That's a fowl one."

"Well, I was winging it."

"You'll egret it."

We haven't been here for a couple of years, not since before I got sick. There are quite a few cars in the parking lot, but we don't see many people because there are several trails through the woods, by the pond, and out to Lake Ontario, so the birdwatchers and families with small children are all spread out. We start on the boardwalk over the pond. We see hundreds of Canada geese, but not much else. Then, by the bridge, Jack spots a large brightly colored duck. He takes a picture of it, to identify it later.

"It's probably an accidental," he says.

"That's not very flattering," Simon remarks.

"Or maybe it escaped from a farm."

We head onto the forest trail. I take out a packet of sunflower seeds from my coat pocket and pass them around.

"What are these?" Simon asks, surprised. "Are these *salted?*"

"They're salted and roasted," I mumble. I'm defensive. I had been the one to run into the No Frills on our way out this morning, while the others waited in the car in the grocery store's parking lot. I grabbed it from the nuts and fruit section at the front. I didn't have time to find the pet section.

"I thought animals needed salt. Don't people set out salt licks for deer?"

"Chickadees are not deer," Jack says firmly.

It turns out Jack and Simon are right—although the chickadees do land on our outstretched palms, they reject the sunflower seeds, even when we peel them. We have better luck with the peanuts I also bought. I love the scritch of their claws on my skin, the whisper of their white breast feathers fluttering in the wind, the almost imperceptible weight on my hand.

CHAPTER TWENTY-NINE

"SEE YOU at Homer's birthday party," Danielle says, as we rise from the table and put on our coats. We've just finished having lunch at a Thai place around the corner from her office.

"What birthday party?" I pause as I'm reaching for my knapsack.

"Oh, the surprise party that..." Her voice trails off when she realizes I know nothing about it. I don't say anything, so she continues to speak.

"...that Danielle Miller is throwing."

I feel a tiny bit better, but not much. At law school twenty years ago I knew Danielle Miller, only slightly, as the "other Danielle," and I would not expect her to include me at any party she was throwing today. Still, if it's for Homer, who is my friend not hers (she doesn't even know him), it doesn't make sense not to include me. I'm hurt.

At this point, I open my eyes. Simon is lying on his side, his head inches from my face, gazing at me intently. His eyes look dark gray in the morning light. I often catch him at this if he wakes up before I do.

"Now I know for sure I'm cured," I announce with satisfaction as if we were already in the middle of a conversation. He raises the one eyebrow not hidden in his pillow.

"Because I'm back to my usual dreams, you know, about, about social faux pas and stuff, stuff I used to fret about." I put my hands together trying to mimic the action Anna does when recounting something socially embarrassing, one hand on top of the other, the thumbs swimming like flippers.

"You know, 'awkward turtle' stuff. Instead of dreaming I was dying, like at Sunnybrook, in the beginning." Before I got sick, my dreams were always about social missteps, mine or other people's. In those days, a bad dream meant one where I hosted a dinner party, and no one liked the meal. Despite the fact that what I had served was squid intestines, I still woke up feeling hurt that Kate, who was one of the guests, hadn't appreciated it. Ever since I told Kate about that dream, whenever she thanks me for anything, she also throws in "And thanks for the squid intestines. They were delicious!"

"If I'm back to these, I must be better," I conclude. "Do you think I should mention it at my appointment this morning?"

"Definitely," says Simon.

"You look like you're going on a date," Simon tells me when I come down the stairs. We're about to leave for my now monthly checkup at the transplant clinic. I'm wearing my new gray-flowered pants, burgundy sleeveless blouse, and black leather jacket.

"I'm celebrating a special occasion," I protest. "It was exactly two years ago today I got my diagnosis."

"Happy anniversary," he says.

"Fine, maybe I said that wrong." I search for another word. "Okay, not celebrating the day, I'm *marking* the day. Is that better?"

Really, it's part of my not-so-secret mission to get my appointments changed from the morning to the afternoon. The sick people, the ones who have to be carefully monitored, come on Monday or Thursday mornings, sometimes both. The well people, who have passed some yet to be specified (to me, that is) hurdle, are in the Monday afternoon clinic and only come every three months to start, and eventually once a year. I asked about it last time, and the resident just smiled sympathetically and said I still had to be monitored closely for graft-versus-host disease. But I know I don't belong with all those sick people, with their bald heads, shaky steps, and IV stands. My strategy this time is to dress so well the doctor will say, "Heavens, you look way too good to be a morning patient, go home this instant and don't come back until Monday afternoon."

"I'm planning to start work in October," I tell the doctor. "That'll be two years post-transplant." I am obsessed with anniversaries. Today is two years post-leukemia diagnosis. In exactly six months, I will hit two years post-stem cell transplant. "I'll be near here, which'll be convenient."

"Yes," he says absently, flipping through my chart to find the latest blood work to show me, "and by then you'll be coming on Monday afternoon, instead of Monday morning."

"Monday *afternoon?*" I might as well have shouted it.

He looks up and smiles. "Yes." He's found the blood work and hands it to me. "You see, your white cell count is good." I look at the closely printed columns of numbers blankly. He points to the right place. "You should know how to read this by now," he chides. I am unabashed. He seems to think I'm making no effort. He doesn't realize how much determination it takes to come through something like this unscathed by knowledge that breeds not understanding, but fear.

I ignore the numbers. Simon's right, I'm busy thinking, my clothes don't matter. What I really need is to hang my work ID card around my neck. I had noticed all the hospital staff do that. Then no one would ever guess I'm a patient. I can't wait for my next appointment.

CHAPTER THIRTY

THE PHONE RINGS in the middle of the afternoon, like it always does. But now my naps are not as sound as they once were. I wake instantly, leap up, and walk around to Simon's side of the bed. We really should move the phone to my side, I think. I'm the only one who ever uses it.

"Hi, it's Judy from Princess Margaret." My stomach flutters. I know exactly who she is. Judy from Princess Margaret Hospital's Donor Services Program, to be precise. I had finally signed the consent form to find out who my donor is. You're allowed to do it once you're one year post-transplant. I got the forms at that time, but then delayed for a few months because, just like all the medical forms I had to sign for the transplant, they listed all the ways things could go wrong. Meeting your donor may lead to unwelcome publicity; you may find you have nothing in common; your donor may not wish to have contact with you; your donor may seek compensation. The latter, especially, hadn't occurred to me.

"I can't imagine people give a cheek swab hoping for compensation," I mused to Simon. "I mean the chance is so remote you're even a match for someone and then it's remote again that the transplant would work. There must be easier ways to make money." Simon agreed, but I kept going. "But what if my donor turns out to be homeless or something? And even if he doesn't ask, or expect, or anything, wouldn't I be morally obligated to give him our house? I mean, he did save my life, even giving everything I have wouldn't repay that."

"If you think you're going to give him our house," Simon said, alarmed, "don't sign the forms!" But I eventually do.

"I have the information you requested" is the next thing Judy says. "Do you have a pencil to write it down?"

"One sec!" I fumble around for something to write with and find a small, wrinkled notepad I'd been using as a coaster for my water glass, but no pencil. I search on Simon's night table and this time I'm successful. "Go ahead." I'm awkwardly cradling the phone between my neck and left shoulder so I can hold the pad down with one hand and write with the other. My stomach is now beyond fluttering and is roiling with excitement. This is it. I carefully write down his name, address, phone number, and email. She repeats everything twice.

"What do you think I should do?" I ask her. "Would it be okay to call? Or should I email first? What do people usually do?"

"Oh, I don't think it matters. Since he gave his phone

number, I'm sure it would be okay to call." I put the phone down. There is no way I can return to my nap. I am too excited.

I tell Simon first.

"We were both wrong," I announce.

"What?"

"You know, you thought Germany, I thought Brampton. He is Indian, I can tell by the name, Jay Sethna, but he lives in New York City, on Staten Island. What do you think? Should I call first or email?"

"You could visit."

"Ohh, I could! New York's not that far." I immediately start planning it. "I could say we were coming to visit New York anyway and wondered if we could meet for a coffee or something. That sounds casual, right? And believable? People from Toronto visit New York all the time, so he wouldn't think I was stalking him or anything, right? Especially if I say my husband and I were planning a trip, that sounds totally normal, doesn't it?"

"Totally."

I tell Jack and Anna.

"Why do you want to visit him?" Jack asks.

I'm dumbfounded. "Are you kidding me? Wouldn't you want to meet the person who saved your life?"

"No!" says Anna. "That would be so awkward."

"Awkward!" I'm amazed. Whose children are these? "We'd have so much to talk about! I want to know every single, little thing about him! No detail about his life would be too small! I want to know everything that happened the day he went to give a cheek swab. What made him go? Was it because of an appeal for someone he knew? And did that person end up getting a match? And—"

"You're going to ask him all that?" Anna looks pained.

"Oh, way more than that." I'm on a roll. "I want to know what went through his mind the moment he got the call that he was a match. I want to know…"

My mother understands. "Of course, in person!" she agrees.

"What kind of name is Sethna, do you know?" I spell it for her.

"I think from Gujarat." She's fairly sure, but not positive. That's the province next to the one I'm from, which makes sense since the people would be close genetically as well.

"If you meet his mother," she urges me, "make sure you tell her thank you from me." She hesitates and clears her throat, "Tell her thank you for raising such a wonderful son."

I hadn't imagined I would be meeting his mother, but you never know. The address had a street number, no apartment number, so it's probably a house. And I was picturing quite a young man. The age range for acceptable donors is seventeen to thirty-five. So maybe he's a university student and the address is his parents' home.

I tell Peter.

"Where are you going to live?" He sounds concerned. I don't know what he's talking about.

"What do you mean, where am I going to live?"

"You were going to give him your house, remember?"

"Oh, that." I shrug. "I have a better idea now. Obviously I can't give him my house, but I was thinking what gift could I give, but it's so hard. I don't know what he would like, and a gift basket would be so cheesy, and a gift certificate, or money, even if it was like a thousand dollars, or something, would cheapen it all, make it all sordid. It would trivialize it all, right?"

Peter doesn't say anything. Does he think I'm being cheap by thinking money would be a cheap gift? I plow on.

"Then I had the best idea. I'm going to give him a photo of the four of us—me, Simon, Jack, Anna—in a pool, in Mexico. And I'll frame it. Wouldn't that be perfect?"

Peter agrees. "That would be perfect."

The family photo idea occurred to me after I spoke at a local high school that was doing a "Get Swabbed" campaign for the stem cell registry. I told the students my story, focusing on how you can help not just one person, but all the people who love that person as well. A girl came up to me afterwards to tell me she liked what I said about how you save a whole family, because, she paused, because her father died of cancer last year. What cancer, I asked because I had to say something. Stomach cancer, she replied, and her eyes suddenly brightened with tears that were reflected in the rush of my own.

I can see it so clearly. He can pull the photo out every once in a while, maybe on a day, or at a time, when things aren't going so well for him, and he can trace our four faces in the blue water, smiling in the sunshine, and tell people, See this family? See how happy they look? This is the family I saved.

Then I have another great idea. I wander into the family room where Simon is watching TV, and inform him that I'm thinking of giving Jay my statue of Ganesh reading a book.

"Because it's my most treasured possession, and I need to give him something priceless, right? Something that money can't buy? What do you think?" Before he can answer, I already have second thoughts. "I don't know if I can actually give it away though. I might miss it too much. It means too much to me."

"If it means that much to you," Simon responds, "then you have to give it." I'm worried it's with my office stuff, all packed away, but luckily I find it easily in one of the boxes a colleague dropped off at home for me, boxes of family photos and Jack and Anna's artwork— things she was worried would get damaged or lost if I left them in the courthouse storage rooms. I tuck it in a bubble wrap pouch, buy a frame for my photo, and I'm ready.

"I have his exact blood!" I tell another friend weeks later. "Literally. Every single cell of my blood is being made by the same stem cells that are making his blood. Isn't that amazing?"

"It is amazing," she responds, intrigued by the possibilities. "Like if your blood was found on a crime scene, the DNA analysis would say it was him! And if they tried to test you, instead of giving a blood sample, you could give a cheek swab, those cells are still yours, right? And then you would get away with it."

That hadn't occurred to me, if it's even true. And I really hope it doesn't occur to him.

I work and rework the email in my mind, right down to the careful wording of the subject line ("RE: Stem cell transplant"). I decide that would be nice and neutral.

Dear Jay,

I am the person whose life you saved. I was diagnosed
with leukemia on April 28, 2014. At that time I was
47 years old, happily married with 11-year-old twins,
and a job I loved. My doctors said that unless I had
a stem cell transplant I only had a 40 percent chance
of surviving. I spent months in hospital undergoing
chemotherapy. But miraculously I found a match in
you and had the stem cell transplant on October 28,
2014. I am almost completely recovered and plan to
return to work this October. My chances of surviving
by that time, two years post transplant, will be 90
percent.

My husband and I are planning a trip to New York
City for a few days in late August or September to
celebrate before I return to work. I would love to
meet you, for an hour or so, for coffee say, while we
are in town. I really hope that will be possible. Are
there days that are better for you? We are flexible
about the timing of our trip.

I look forward to meeting you,

Manjusha

He emails me back immediately and it's like correspond-
ing with someone I already know. He's thrilled I'm visiting
and tells me to come anytime. He tells me that the moment

he got the phone call, more than a year after the transplant, telling him it was successful and I was doing well, was the most gratifying moment of his life. We email back and forth asking each other questions. I struggle with using the words "thank you" in the emails and decide in the end not to use them at all, because I don't want to trivialize them or ever sign off with the "thanks, Manjusha" that I use in almost every email I send, work or personal. I want to save those words for when we meet, so they will be fresh.

The night before we leave, I'm too tense to sleep. I lie down for only a few seconds before leaping out of bed because I forgot to tell Jack something. I can see from under his door that his light is still on, so I knock, and then enter. He props himself up so he can see me from his top bunk where he's reading. He puts his book down; the earbuds from his iPod dangle from one ear. He looks at me questioningly.

"I forgot to tell you. You know those papers you asked me to sign for your trip? I checked and they're not due until next week, so I'll do it when we get back from New York. Okay?"

"Okay." He returns to his book and I close the door and return to bed.

Minutes later I'm back at his door. His light is off now, but I figure he can't be asleep yet. I knock again.

"What?" The room is dark, but I can almost make him out.

"I realized we were talking about you starting to volunteer at Cubs tomorrow, but September 28 is actually next Wednesday, not tomorrow, tomorrow's the 21st. So I wanted to let you know it's next week, not tomorrow like we thought."

"Oh, yeah, right."

"Good night."

"Good night."

I'm in bed for almost an hour before I realize I better cross off the line about Jack being at Cubs from the note I left for my mother on the kitchen counter. I go downstairs and amend the schedule.

At 3 a.m. I'm back in the kitchen, this time to cut the tight shrink wrap off the cheddar. It's always hard to cut it off an unopened wedge. Anna will be making her own lunch tomorrow and I don't want her to cut her hand. I rewrap the cheddar in plastic wrap and return it to the fridge.

It's too overwhelming to think about meeting Jay, so I continue to think about cheese until finally it's 5 a.m. and time to get up to catch our flight.

When we finally make it to Central Park, where we have planned to meet Jay, we have just enough time to grab a quick lunch before our meeting. We get a couple of hot dogs from one of the vendors lined up outside the entrance and carry them carefully into the park; I'm wearing a white shirt and don't want to show up for this momentous meeting covered in mustard and ketchup. We are halfway through our lunch when I notice, from reading the sign on a hot dog cart inside the park, that we have been charged double the usual price. I'm assuming it was because the vendor could tell we were tourists, with our backpacks, and especially with Simon's British accent. Simon's philosophical about it. "I guess we've learned a valuable lesson," he says. But I'm furious.

"It's the principle, not the nine dollars," I repeat, as I insist we march back to the vendors.

I can't believe it. The cart we got the hot dogs from is

gone. Even though it's only half an hour later, it's been replaced by a cart selling Popsicles. I approach several nearby vendors to ask if they've seen the hot dog cart that was right beside the book kiosk. One vendor is particularly sympathetic, or possibly worried I'm about to embark on an exposé of Central Park hot dog vendors. He brings out a battered sandwich board listing prices to show me that his own business is honest. "Next time go to the police!" he tells me. "It's bad for the rest of us too when this happens."

Simon waits, at first patiently, and then, not so patiently, for me to focus. "We're going to be late to meet Jay," he warns me.

"Let me just ask one more person," I say, "and maybe that person over there too if they know where that cart went." No one knows. It's very difficult. The sun is so hot and it's all too much. The buskers that were sitting near us move farther down to a bench that's in the shade. My eyes are burning from lack of sleep. I was so eager in anticipating this day; now it's here, I feel slightly sick.

I give up on finding the vendor and we re-enter the park. I perk up when we reach the pond with the remote-controlled sailboats. I recognize them even though I've never seen them before. I realize this is where Stuart Little raced his sailboat. I hadn't known until now it was an actual thing, not just a scene in the story about the famous mouse. Finally we're at our meeting point, the Alice in Wonderland statue. It's beautiful, shining in the sun, and the White Rabbit, the Mad Hatter, and the dormouse are there too. In a real garden. Look how far I've come, I want to tell Alice, from those flowers in the hospital's glass garden. Simon and I sit and watch

while people stroll by stopping for photos. We forgot to bring
our camera. We switch to a shady bench.

Then I see a young Indian man walking quickly toward
us and suddenly he's right in front of me and we're hugging
and he's sobbing and for some reason I'm laughing, but I can't
say anything. He's late, he eventually explains, because he
walked in the wrong direction from the subway station.

I'm usually chatty, but I find it difficult to speak. I was
saving "thank you" for this moment, but I can't say it. The
words are used up, too meager, too ordinary. I've said them
a hundred times today already, to the shuttle bus driver for
dropping us off at the airport, to the flight attendant for giving me a bottle of water, to the woman crossing the street
with us for telling us which way was west, even to the vendor
who handed me our nine-dollar hot dogs.

I'll save it for later, I think, when we're at his house, with
everyone gathered around. He had invited us to Staten Island
to meet his family. It'll be better there, I decide, it'll be special, like a speech. So I don't say much now, I just ask him
questions. I'm starving for every detail of his journey. How he
was in his last month of law school when he got the call, how
he thought it was a telemarketer at first, because he didn't
remember the name of the blood services. It had been seven
years since he'd given a cheek swab at a Gujarati conference,
in response to a plea by a member of their community. He
was twenty years old at the time, and he'd casually given the
swab as he was heading out for a drink with friends. Luckily,
there was no lineup, or he may not even have paused to do it.

When he finally understood what they were calling
about, that he was a match for someone, he had only one

question: "Are there any other matches?" And when they said, "No, you're the only one we found," he said, "I'll do it." Before they explained anything about the process, about what it would entail, even when he mistakenly believed it would involve an operation, he still said yes immediately.

"I'm scared of doctors," he says sheepishly, "so I never go, and then I had to do all these tests to see if I was healthy, an EKG and stuff, so I was glad to find out I was." But then he was annoyed when, in the week or so before the transplant, he got not just one call, but several, to confirm he was really willing to go through with it, that he hadn't changed his mind.

"I said I would do it!" he remembers telling them, thinking they shouldn't be questioning his commitment, and also thinking that their repeated checks would scare people by making them believe it was a bigger deal than they had thought it would be. "I thought they were like inviting people to back out, it didn't make sense," he says.

Then they explained to him that it was because I was about to start the chemo and radiation treatments to wipe out my immune system before the transplant. If he changed his mind after I started those treatments, I would die, because not only would I not be getting his immune system, I would no longer have mine. He said they told him it had happened, a related donor had changed his mind the very day of the transplant, and the patient died. They wanted to impress upon him that if he was going to change his mind, now was the time to do it.

But far from changing his mind he never faltered. He says the daily injections the week before the donation hurt for a few seconds, but the donation itself, though it took a few hours, didn't hurt at all. They kept him supplied with juice and cookies and a courier was right there, waiting to take the bag the second it was finished. "The nurse there asked me if I knew how lucky I was," he said. I am surprised to hear that. Then he explains, "She said because lots of people give a cheek swab and don't match with anyone. And I thought, yeah, I'm lucky. This is the biggest thing I've ever done, that I'll ever do."

"And it worked," I marvel.

"Oh, I knew it would work," he says, sounding utterly certain.

"What do you mean, you knew?"

"So many things had to happen," he explains. "I've never even given blood before. That was the only time I ever gave a cheek swab. And the time of the procedure I was between law school and working, I was completely free. I made the donation in the same hospital I was born in. If all that worked, it meant the transplant just had to work."

The lesser stars aligned as well. We're both in law; we both love the same television series (*The Wire*, *Breaking Bad*, *Making a Murderer*); we both worry about the words we use; we both have a terrible sense of direction. On our way to his home, he got turned around at the subway station by the ferry docks.

"There's no sign," I say to Simon, sympathizing with Jay's confusion.

"Well, the ferry is probably by the water," Simon points out, unsympathetically, as we retrace our steps and head toward the river.

At his home, we meet his parents and his grandmother whom he lives with. They are all so happy to see me, like I'm the special one. I can't believe I made it this far, and they can't believe I'm here. I want to say my thank you now, but I feel overwhelmed and underprepared. I decide really I should wait until his fiancée and his brother and sister-in-law arrive; they are coming directly from work. Instead, I hand his mother a package from my mother containing five kinds of Indian sweets she has made (the number you make when you're celebrating) and a letter. His mother starts to read the letter in front of us, but has to put it away for later because it makes her tear up.

"His brother gave a cheek swab that day also," his mother tells me on a more cheerful note, "and oh, he was so disappointed when Jay turned out to be a match instead of him. 'Why didn't I match?' he wanted to know. Why Jay?"

His grandmother says something in Gujarati and his mother translates. "She says Jay must have taken something from you in a former life and now he's giving it back."

Jay's mother puts the photo I gave Jay on an end table with a cluster of other photos of engagements and weddings and vacations. She puts my Ganesh on a shrine at one end of the living room; he fits right in, as there are at least a dozen other Ganesh figures spread out across the table. But they are softer featured and all white; he is small and precise and dark gray, intent upon his book. I feel a pang, which I ignore.

Jay tells me blood services sent him a thank you card after the transplant with some movie tickets, which he thought was nice. And today, the exact day we're meeting, he got an email inviting him to participate in one of those runs to raise money. He hands me his phone to read the message, because he's so amazed by the timing. I murmur at the coincidence of it all, but really I'm cringing when I scroll down to where they tell him that, because he's a donor, he'll get ten dollars off the registration fee. Really, ten dollars? Suddenly I'm upset. Nothing, nothing, nothing is enough.

The rest of the family eventually arrives, but in the bustle of introductions I miss my moment to make a speech, and now it's time to eat, so I decide to wait until after dinner.

I learn that Jay's in the process of being admitted to the New York bar. He wants to go into criminal law, to be a public defender. His fiancée laughs when I mention wonderingly that he seems too good to be true. She describes how they met at a conference two years ago at which he had sung the American and the Indian national anthems. "I was sitting beside him," she tells me, "and people kept coming by saying, great singing, congratulations on law school, hey we heard you saved someone's life, and I was thinking who *is* this?"

"Hold September 1, 2, and 3," his mother tells me. "For the wedding. And your children and your parents, your whole family, must come." I smile and nod and think a Labor Day weekend of festivities with 400 people we've never met would be a pretty accurate depiction of Simon's idea of hell. But then it hits me, who Jay is. He's my blood brother. Literally.

If you actually think about bloodlines, blood relations, blood being thicker than water, then we are closer to each other than to anyone else in our families. I turn over my hands and look down at my pink palms. The blood that my heart is pumping every second to my fingertips, to every part of my body, is the same as the blood that is flowing through his veins right now. Every single cell of my blood comes from his stem cells, the same stem cells his own blood is coming from.

I look over at him. We're now at the end of the evening; we're done eating, we're done talking; he has brought down the family's harmonium to the living room and is playing and singing an Indian classical song while his brother accompanies him on the tabla and his mother and grandmother tilt their heads and call out in soft bursts of appreciation.

I tilt my own head and glance at Simon. He's on the sofa and he's looking at me and smiling. And I know he knows. Of course we will go to the wedding. Jay is my brother. His family opening their arms to me was much more than Indian hospitality; they did it with full hearts, welcoming a daughter, a granddaughter, a sister. I had been looking forward to this trip as the endpoint of my ordeal, my chance to thank the person who saved my life. Turns out I haven't ended anything, I've added another whole family to my life.

He drops us off at the ferry docks, narrowly avoiding several collisions in the process, honking at every driver in front of us who has the temerity to slow down for a yellow light. We benefit from the breakneck speed, and manage to catch the ferry seconds before the gates close. The New York City skyline glitters against the blue-black night. The light of the Statue of Liberty's torch is like a star, and I'm busy planning what to give him for his birthday (just two months away), what to give him for his wedding, even what to get for the birth of his future child, when I realize I never did say thank you.

"Don't worry," Simon says. "I said it."

"Not just for dinner right? But for actually—"
"Yes," Simon confirms. "Not just for dinner."

I'm going to steal a line from Simon to end, which should not surprise anyone because all the best lines in this book are his. It's something he's been saying to me starting in Rome, and almost every day since; yes, even through all this cancer stuff. But I'm not remotely ashamed by my theft, because the words make much more sense coming from me.

"Will you tell me now? How did I get to be so lucky?"

THE END

EPILOGUE

SAVITRI SITS under the spreading branches of a banyan tree, Satyavan's head in her lap. Her fingers are raking softly through his hair, as light as the breeze that lifts the ends of her own unbraided locks that ripple down her back. But the only breath that joins the breeze is hers.

"It is time."

She doesn't have to look up to know who has spoken. After all, she has spent the last three days with no sleep closing her eyes, no food or water passing her lips, as upright as the trees she stood among, with prayers as silent as theirs. But still he came, just as she knew he would.

Her lips press tightly together, but otherwise she doesn't stir as Yama bends down between the backswept horns of the wild water buffalo he rides and effortlessly lifts up her husband's body and drapes it in front of him. She doesn't even look up until the god of death is almost out of sight, his dark ox and darker skin melting into the night.

Though he would never admit it, being a god and all, he is relieved. He thought for sure he would have trouble with her. She is famous; the only child of a king who prayed to the sun god for years, literally years, for a son. The sun god, impressed with the king's steadfastness, said, "You have been so faithful I will grant you more than what you seek. I will grant you not a son, but a daughter whose capacity for devotion will one day match your own. Trust me, it will be better this way." If the king was disappointed he hid it well, loved his daughter warmly, and indulged her in every way. He even let her leave to search for a husband herself when she grew up to be so beautiful and so pure that no man dared approach to ask for her hand in marriage.

And one day she finds her soulmate, in a forest—a young man perfect in every way, bold and handsome, brilliant and loving, son of a blind hermit king. But there's a catch, as you knew there would be. He is doomed to die in exactly one year. My mother says it's because his parents made their own deal at his birth. When they fasted and prayed for a child, they were given a choice: an ordinary child who lives a long but ordinary life, or a perfect son who dies young, and they went with the latter.

Savitri's father, not thrilled with the idea of a doomed son-in-law, tries to dissuade his daughter. "Are you sure about this?" he asks. "I know a king who knows a king whose youngest son is supposed to have a great personality. I could send out some messengers." But she is sure. She gives up her silks and jewels and goes to live in the forest with Satyavan and his exiled parents. And they live in happiness for every day of that year.

Yama stiffens. He thinks he hears something. He pauses. Yes, there it is again, the soft crackle of footsteps through the leaves on the forest floor. He looks over his shoulder. Savitri is following him. He sighs. This is more like what he was expecting.

"Stay here," he says. "This is your home. You can return with no regrets. You were a good and loving wife."

"It is a wife's dharma," she says, "to go wherever her husband goes, as you of all gods must know."

She has him there, he must acknowledge, however reluctantly. His full name is Yamadharma after all, for he is also responsible for upholding dharma, the eternal law of the cosmos inherent in the very nature of things, the law that even the gods have to obey.

"Your words are music to my ears," he says with gritted teeth. "You are right. For displaying this wisdom I will grant you one boon, anything you ask—"

She immediately opens her mouth.

"—except your husband's life!" he adds hastily, before she can speak.

She is unperturbed and has another request at the ready. "I ask that you restore the sight to my father-in-law's eyes."

"Done," says Yama, happy that she has asked for something so simple. "He will be marveling at the beauties of the forest canopy before you have time to return to his side."

"Oh, I'm not going home."

"What do you mean?" Yama cries. "You can't follow me.

My kingdom is far away. You will tire long before we reach it."

"I won't be tired if I'm with my husband," Savitri persists. "I will go where he goes. And one never tires in the company of gods; walking with gods is never futile."

"Your words are water to my thirsty soul," he mutters. He is annoyed and flattered at the same time. "I will grant you a second boon. And before you ask, the same rules apply."

"I ask that you grant my father a hundred sons so his name will live on."

"Done," says Yama and spurs his buffalo to go. It's not like Satyavan's is the only soul he has to collect before the night is through. Several hours go by and when his buffalo stops to drink at a glistening stream, Yama dismounts to stretch his legs. And there behind him, at a respectful distance, but there against his express directive nonetheless, is Savitri.

"Seriously?" he asks. "What part of 'go home' did you not understand? Go back. You have walked much too far."

"Too far from what?" Savitri demands. Her back is still straight and her feet, though bare, are unbruised by the tree roots and fallen twigs she has been walking over for uncounted winding miles. "How can I be far from anywhere if I am near my husband?"

Yama laughs. She is beginning to grow on him, this girl who won't go away. He was a man first, before he became a god. The first man who ever died, in fact, which is why he gets to preside over all who die after him. So he can just about remember what it was like to live and then to die. He is pretty sure he did not want to die.

"One more boon," he says, still laughing.

"I ask for a hundred sons for myself."

He stops laughing but he is not angry. Far from it. She has surprised him. She has not only impressed him with her devotion, she has outsmarted him with her wit. He cannot grant the final boon he promised her without also returning her husband. He tugs Satyavan's body off the buffalo and sets him down to stand beside his wife. And, passing from Yama's cold hands to Savitri's warm ones, Satyavan revives, and Yama rides on.

And every thousand years or so, if a wife, or a husband, is as devoted as Savitri was to Satyavan, if they follow their spouse almost to the gates of the Kingdom of Death itself, which I happen to know is situated somewhere between Cancer Ward 2 and the ICU at Sunnybrook Hospital, they can win them back. They don't have to be perfect; they don't even have to fight. They just have to be there for every single step. We make bargains every day whether we believe in the gods we make them with or not. In fact, it's the gods you don't believe in that can really fuck you up. And the only thing that can save you in the end is love.

That last line sounds poetic, but it makes me uneasy. I want to delete it because, while I feel that I was saved by love—from family, from friends, from a stranger—there are many others who are just as beloved but who still do not make it. At first, I'm depressed, thinking it's so sad to have to admit that love can't actually save us. But then I think, wait! Doesn't that make love *more* amazing, as opposed to less? More touching?

We can't always save the people we love with our love, and yet...and yet we go ahead and love them anyway.

We hold our breath in wonder, so we can hear them breathe.

THE END
(Really.)

ACKNOWLEDGMENTS

This book was a lifeline thrown to me by my friend Peter Nosalik, who formed our writers' group at the darkest time of my life. When I just served up snacks instead of stories for the first few meetings, his stern admonishment of "Less baking, more writing!" kick-started this book. A heartfelt thank you to him and the other members, Melany Franklin, Melanie Hazell, and Karyn O'Neill, for their enthusiastic support and insightful criticism. I am also deeply indebted to my husband, Simon, and friend Nancy Naylor for their detailed and thoughtful readings of my manuscript, and to my publisher Margie Wolfe at Second Story Press for believing in me from the beginning. And really, it started with my mother. Her passion for literature and her commitment to Nachiket Children's Libraries, which provides books to children in rural India, taught me that a book is just as likely to save you as anything else.

If I listed all the friends, neighbors, colleagues, and family members who leapt up to help me in so many ways through this crisis, this acknowledgment section would be as long as the book itself. So, to those who are named in the book, and to the countless others who are not, thank you. I always knew I had great friends, but I did not know until now, just how many, and just how great.

Thank you also to the incredible doctors, nurses, and all the other staff that make up Canada's amazing health care system. They made me so proud and so grateful to be Canadian.

Finally, thank you to Jay, for giving me life.

And thank you to Simon, Jack, and Anna, for making my life worth living.

ABOUT THE AUTHOR

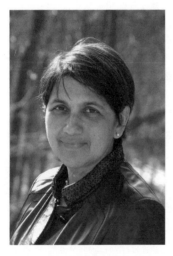

MANJUSHA PAWAGI has a law degree from the University of Toronto and a journalism degree from Stanford University. She has worked as a reporter for CBC Radio in Charlottetown, P.E.I., and The Associated Press in St. Louis, Mo.; and as a lawyer for the Children's Aid Society of Toronto and the Office of the Children's Lawyer. She was appointed to the Ontario Court of Justice in 2009 and she is currently a family and youth court judge in Toronto. She is the author of a best-selling children's book, *The Girl Who Hated Books*, which has been translated into more than a dozen languages and made into an award-winning animated short by the National Film Board of Canada. She lives in Toronto with her husband Simon, children Jack and Anna, and a pet lizard who prefers to remain anonymous.

12/23